LABORATORY PROCEDURES

for Pharmacy Technicians

LABORATORY PROCEDURES

for Pharmacy Technicians

Jahangir Moini, MD, MPH, CPhT
Professor and Former Director, Allied
Health Sciences

Pharmacy Technician Program
Everest University
Melbourne, Florida

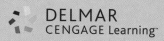

DELMAR
CENGAGE Learning™

Australia • Brazil • Japan • Korea • Mexico • Singapore • Spain • United Kingdom • United States

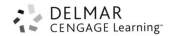

**Laboratory Procedures
for Pharmacy Technicians**
Jahangir Moini, MD, MPH, CPhT

Vice President, Career and
Professional Editorial: Dave Garza

Director of Learning Solutions:
Matthew Kane

Acquisitions Editor: Tari Broderick

Managing Editor: Marah Bellegarde

Senior Product Manager:
Darcy M. Scelsi

Editorial Assistant: Ian Lewis

Vice President, Career and
Professional Marketing: Jennifer McAvey

Marketing Manager: Kristin McNary

Marketing Coordinator: Erica Ropitzky

Production Director: Carolyn Miller

Production Manager: Andrew Crouth

Senior Art Director: Jack Pendleton

For product information and technology assistance, contact us at
Cengage Learning Customer & Sales Support, 1-800-354-9706

For permission to use material from this text or product,
submit all requests online at **cengage.com/permissions**
Further permissions questions can be emailed to
permissionrequest@cengage.com

Library of Congress Control Number: 2009929658

ISBN-13: 978-1-4180-7394-7

ISBN 10: 1-4180-7394-6

Delmar
5 Maxwell Drive
Clifton Park, NY 12065-2919
USA

Cengage Learning is a leading provider of customized learning solutions with office locations around the globe, including Singapore, the United Kingdom, Australia, Mexico, Brazil, and Japan. Locate your local office at:
international.cengage.com/region

Cengage Learning products are represented in Canada by Nelson Education, Ltd.

To learn more about Delmar, visit **www.cengage.com/delmar**

Purchase any of our products at your local college store or at our preferred online store **www.ichapters.com**

Notice to the Reader

Publisher does not warrant or guarantee any of the products described herein or perform any independent analysis in connection with any of the product information contained herein. Publisher does not assume, and expressly disclaims, any obligation to obtain and include information other than that provided to it by the manufacturer. The reader is expressly warned to consider and adopt all safety precautions that might be indicated by the activities described herein and to avoid all potential hazards. By following the instructions contained herein, the reader willingly assumes all risks in connection with such instructions. The publisher makes no representations or warranties of any kind, including but not limited to, the warranties of fitness for particular purpose or merchantability, nor are any such representations implied with respect to the material set forth herein, and the publisher takes no responsibility with respect to such material. The publisher shall not be liable for any special, consequential, or exemplary damages resulting, in whole or part, from the readers' use of, or reliance upon, this material.

Printed in the United States of America
1 2 3 4 5 6 7 13 12 11 10 09

Dedication

This book is dedicated to
The living memory of my father and
my sister Pari,
My loving and caring family:
Mother, wife, and daughters.

Contents

Part 1   **Theory Review and Procedures**

Section I   **General Concepts**

Section II   Nonsterile Compounding Products

Chapter 4: Equipment and Supplies for
Nonsterile Compounding. 64

Section III Sterile Compounding Products

Part 2   Self-Evaluation

Appendices

Preface

INTRODUCTION

Compounding is one of the major tasks of pharmacy technicians. Nonsterile compounding is one of the most challenging activities in the pharmacy and pharmacy technicians must have specific education and training in this area. This textbook provides students with hands-on, step-by-step procedures that they will find essential for laboratory work. Prior study of anatomy, physiology, chemistry, and pathology is helpful in understanding the skills that are taught in this textbook. Key principles of laboratory activities are described in this text, as well as explanation of equipment and the laboratory environment.

ORGANIZATION OF CONTENT

This book is organized into two parts, "Theory Review and Procedures," and "Self-Evaluation." The first part consists of three sections, "General Concepts," "Nonsterile Compounding Products," and "Sterile Compounding Products," which collectively contain eleven chapters. The Self-Evaluation part of this book features one test for each of the three sections found in Part One. Following Part Two is an answer key, appendices, a glossary, and an index.

FEATURES

Each chapter contains an outline of the key topics, objectives that the student must be able to meet upon completion of the reading, and a list of key terms (which are **bolded** in the chapter text). Overviews serve to introduce the student to the key concepts of the chapter. Figures serve to accurately illustrate chapter principles and related information. Accurate tables focus on essential information that must be fully understood in order to master each chapter's content. Step-by-step procedures are listed which correspond to the figures to show equipment, materials to be handled, and actual tasks. Special "Alert" features are distributed throughout each chapter, highlighting key information. Chapter summaries serve to reinforce the chapter content and focus on key ideas from the text. At the end of each chapter, review questions are given that help students to test the knowledge they have gained from their reading. The questions are given in a variety of formats to encourage more complete comprehension. Lab activities are listed so that students may practice their skills. Book and Web site references are given so that students may seek out additional information to complement their studies. The answer key to each chapter's review questions is also provided.

INSTRUCTOR RESOURCES

This book is accompanied by an Instructor Resources CD containing:

- Critical Thinking Activities.
- Skills Checklists for Laboratory Procedures.
- Image Library.
- Material and Equipment Lists.
- Grading Rubrics.

Acknowledgments

The author would like to acknowledge the following individuals for their time and efforts in aiding him with their contributions to this book.

Andrew Cameron, CPhT
GE Health Care
Melbourne, Florida

Michael Edwards, PharmD
Corporate Director of Pharmacy
Health First
Melbourne, Florida

Norman Tomaka, CRPh, LHCRM
President and Chairman of the Executive Board
Florida Pharmacy Association
and Pharmacist Consultant
Melbourne, Florida

Greg Vadimsky, Pharmacy Technician
Melbourne, Florida

Lee Anna Obos, B.S.

Melinda Reed, B.S. M.B.A.

Aimee Strang, PharmD, B.C.P.S.

REVIEWERS

Denise Anderson, CPhT
United Education Institute
Fontana, California

William J. Havins, BUS, CPhT
Central New Mexico Community College
Albuquerque, New Mexico

Paul Lee, CPhT
CVS
Mechanicsville, Virginia

Lia Mays, CPhT
Everest College
Arlington, Texas

Phil D. Penrod, Jr., BS, AA.AA, CPhT
Corinthian Colleges
Tampa, Florida

Betty Stahl, PharmD
ASA Institute
Brooklyn, New York

Leslie Vandergrift, CPhT
Specialty Pharmacy
Melbourne, Florida

About the Author

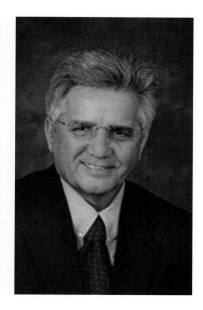

Dr. Moini was assistant professor at Tehran University School of Medicine for 9 years teaching medical and allied health students, and is a professor and former director (for 15 years) of allied health programs at Everest University. In 2000, Dr. Moini established, for the first time, the associate degree program for pharmacy technicians at Everest University's Melbourne campus. For 5 years, he was the director of the pharmacy technician program. He also established several other new allied health programs for Everest University. As a physician and instructor for the past 35 years, he believes that pharmacy technicians should be skillful with various types of compounding and have confidence in their duties and responsibilities in order to prevent medication errors.

Dr. Moini is actively involved in teaching and helping students to prepare for service in various health professions, including the roles of pharmacy technicians, medical assistants, and nurses. He worked with the Brevard County Health Department as an epidemiologist and health educator consultant for 18 years, offering continuing education courses and keeping nurses up-to-date on the latest developments related to pharmacology, medications errors, immunizations, and other important topics. He has been an internationally published author of various allied health books since 1999.

THEORY REVIEW AND PROCEDURES

1

GENERAL CONCEPTS

Safety in the Workplace

OBJECTIVES

Upon completion of this chapter, the student should be able to:

1. Identify the two infections that the Bloodborne Pathogens Standard was created to reduce.
2. Describe Standard Precautions.
3. Explain the Occupational Safety and Health Administration (OSHA) Standards.
4. Discuss reduction of exposure to radiation.
5. Describe the elements required for fire.
6. List five measures to prevent fire.
7. Describe the types of information contained in Material Safety Data Sheets (MSDS).
8. Define ergonomics as related to the workplace.

GLOSSARY

Barrier precautions – Precautions used to minimize the risk of exposure to blood and body fluids; this includes personal protective equipment.

Biohazard symbol – Symbols used to designate biologic materials that may be infective, and can possibly threaten humans or the environment.

Engineering controls – Devices that isolate or remove the bloodborne pathogen hazard from the workplace.

Ergonomic – The applied science of equipment design, intended to maximize productivity by reducing operator fatigue and discomfort.

Exposure control plan – A set of written procedures for the treatment of persons exposed to biohazards or similar chemically harmful materials.

Hazard communication plan – The application of warning labels that signify different types of hazardous chemicals.

Hazardous waste – A substance that is potentially damaging to living organisms and the environment.

Material Safety Data Sheet (MSDS) – Written or printed material concerning a hazardous chemical that includes information on the chemical's identity, as well as physical and chemical characteristics.

Occupational Safety and Health Administration (OSHA) – A Department of Labor agency that is responsible for ensuring safety at work and a healthful work environment.

Personal protective equipment (PPE) – Specialized clothing or equipment worn to protect against health and safety standards.

Sanitization – Cleaning the environment to reduce the number of pathogenic microorganisms.

Standard Precautions – A set of guidelines for infection control.

Work practice controls – Precautionary measures that are taken to reduce possible exposure to bloodborne pathogens by altering the way a procedure is performed.

OVERVIEW

Safety is a basic need in all professions, regardless of the work setting. Pharmacies and laboratories are responsible for providing employees with a safe work environment. This incorporates safety precautions, infection control practices, and hygiene assistance.

Employees must know and understand the hazards that exist in the work environment in order to protect themselves and others. This knowledge greatly reduces the potential risk of work-related injuries. Pharmacy technicians, like other health care providers, must be knowledgeable and aware of the risks for injury in the workplace.

OCCUPATIONAL SAFETY AND HEALTH ADMINISTRATION (OSHA)

In 1970, the Occupational Safety and Health Act was passed to ensure safe and healthful working conditions in the United States. This national health and safety law established the **Occupational Safety and Health Administration (OSHA)**, a part of the Department of Labor. OSHA establishes safety regulations for employers and monitors compliance. Workplaces must be kept free from recognized hazards that may cause serious injury or death. Employees are required to abide by all the safety and health standards that apply to their jobs. Table 1-1 outlines some of the safety practices to which a pharmacy technician should be alert in the workplace.

TABLE 1-1 Safety Guidelines for the Pharmacy Technician

- Observe warning labels on biohazard containers and equipment.
- Minimize splashing, spraying, and splattering of drops of potentially harmful chemicals or infectious materials. Splattering of blood onto skin or mucous membranes is a proven mode of transmission of hepatitis B virus.
- Bandage any breaks or lesions on the hands before gloving.
- If exposed body surfaces come in contact with body fluids, scrub with soap and water as soon as possible. If the eyes are exposed to body fluids, flush with water, preferably using an eyewash station.
- Do not recap, bend, or break contaminated needles and other sharps.
- Use hemostats to attach and remove scalpel blades from handles.
- Do not use mouth pipetting or suck blood or other harmful chemicals through tubing.
- Decontaminate contaminated test materials before reprocessing or place in impervious bags and dispose of according to policy.
- Do not keep food and drink in refrigerators, freezers, shelves, or cabinets, or on countertops where blood or other potentially hazardous chemical materials could be present.

OSHA provides information, education, research, and training, as well as authorized enforcement of its standards. It regulates all workplaces by enforcing the proper removal of hazards, as well as the implementation of fire safety plans and emergency plans. Employees who may be exposed to physical hazards, biological hazards, and chemical dangers must receive information and training about safe work practices designed to reduce these dangers.

OSHA regulations require employers to follow certain steps to ensure the safety and health of their employees. These regulations are intended to ensure that employers provide a safe and healthy workplace for employees. OSHA may inspect both private and public workplaces in order to ensure that all protocols and guidelines are being followed.

OSHA STANDARDS

Many hazards exist in pharmaceutical settings over which OSHA has the power to enforce safety standards and to cite or discipline agencies that do not comply with these standards (Bending, 2000). OSHA regulations as applicable to the pharmacy industry are comprised of two standards:

- The Hazard Communication Standard
- The Bloodborne Pathogen Standard

Additional general industry standards regulated by OSHA that are also applicable to the pharmacy include fire safety, emergency plans, environmental pollution, noise reduction, latex allergies, work-related musculoskeletal injuries, exposure to chemotherapeutic agents, ergonomics, and workplace violence.

The Hazard Communication Standard

The purpose of the Hazard Communication Standard is to ensure that employers and employees are provided information on all hazardous chemicals that may be encountered in the workplace. Many hazards that exist in the health care work environment can cause injury to employees. In many workplaces, including the pharmacy, chemicals (including chlorine bleach, cleaning supplies, disinfectants, and other products) can cause serious injury if handled or contained improperly. Chemicals pose a risk to employees by direct absorption through the skin, ingestion, inhalation, entry through the mucous membranes, or entry through a break in the skin. Electrical equipment, pharmacy instruments, and glassware can all be hazards if they are improperly used.

These hazards must be communicated in a plan that specifies labeling requirements, requires the use and maintenance of Material Data Safety Sheets (MSDS), and outlines an employee training program.

The Hazard Communication Plan

Employers must write and maintain a **hazard communication plan** for the workplace. This plan should address the responsibilities of labeling hazardous materials, maintaining a list of all hazardous materials, keeping MSDS forms up to date, outlining the training requirements and employee responsibilities toward training, and outlining an exposure control plan. This plan must be available for all employees. Safety signs should be posted appropriately throughout the pharmacy. They serve as a constant reminder to employees and ensure safe work practices.

OSHA requires employers to inform their employees of the following:

- The location of Material Safety Data Sheets.
- The hazards existing in the workplace and where they are located in the building or buildings.
- The location of hazard-related information.
- How to read and understand hazard signs and chemical labels.
- What type of personal protective equipment must be worn while working with hazardous chemicals and where this equipment is stored.
- How to manage spills and where cleaning equipment is stored.

Inventory of Products

All products in a workplace that are potentially hazardous must be identified as such. A list of these hazardous materials must be a part of the hazard communication plan. This list serves as an inventory of products and an MSDS must be maintained for all products identified on the list. Common materials found in the pharmacy that may be hazardous include: inks, oil products, cleaners, glues, toner, silicone lubricants, controlled substances, radiopharmaceuticals, gases, and alcohols. Some drugs considered hazardous by OSHA include the following: altretamine, bleomycin, cisplatin, dactinomycin, ethinyl estradiol, fluorouracil, ganciclovir, hydroxyurea, interferon-A, lomustine, methotrexate, nafarelin, plicamycin, ribavirin, streptozocin, tamoxifen, uracil mustard, vinblastine, and zidovudine.

Labeling Hazardous Materials

All products in the workplace must be properly labeled by the product manufacturer. The labels must be legible and intact. The label should identify the chemical, list warnings about hazards, and include the name and address of the manufacturer. Hazardous products must be kept in their original containers. Their original labels must be intact and legible (Figure 1-1). All chemicals in health care facilities must be kept in locked cupboards.

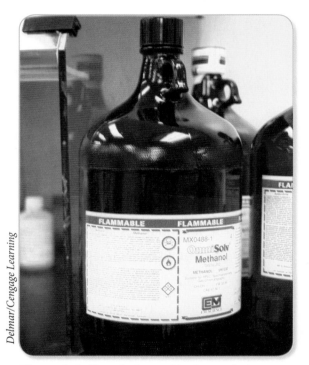

Delmar/Cengage Learning

Figure 1-1 Chemicals used in the workplace must be clearly and accurately labeled.

Material Safety Data Sheet

The **Material Safety Data Sheet (MSDS)** is a document that outlines the structure of a chemical substance and identifies the potential hazards of that substance. This document must supply the chemical and common name, chemical composition, characteristics of the substance, hazards of the substance, guidelines for safe handling and disposal of the substance, and guidelines for emergency procedures. Appendix A provides a sample of an MSDS sheet. Employers must maintain up-to-date and accurate MSDS records for each hazardous chemical in their facility. The employer must make this information available to employees.

Training Programs

Employers must provide training to employees upon hire regarding the hazards that may be encountered in the workplace. Any time new hazards are introduced, additional training on those hazards must be provided to all employees. Accurate records must be maintained documenting the training that has been provided and the employees' acknowledgement of completion of the training.

The Bloodborne Pathogen Standard

The Bloodborne Pathogen Standard is intended to reduce occupational-related cases of HIV and HBV infections among health care workers. It covers all employees who can be "reasonably anticipated" to come into contact with blood, body fluids, and other potentially infectious materials. It seeks to limit exposure to these bloodborne pathogens.

Exposure Control Plan

An **exposure control plan** must outline how a particular workplace is going to handle potential hazards from exposure to blood, body fluids, or other potentially infectious materials. The plan must be reviewed and updated annually, and training on the plan must be given to all employees. The employer must elicit input from the employees who are at risk when making revisions to the plan. The plan must be available to employees at all times.

Exposure Determination

A part of the exposure control plan is to define the risk of the employees. There are generally three levels of risk: (I) exposure is anticipated when normally performing the job (physicians, nurses); (II) only occasional exposure is anticipated when normally performing the job (pharmacist, pharmacy technician); (III) no exposure is anticipated when normally performing the job.

Standard Precautions

Standard Precautions are those methods that can be implemented and used to minimize the risk of exposure to employees. These methods of control include hand hygiene; use of personal protective equipment; standards for handling sharps, cleanup of spills, disposal and disinfection of equipment, handling of soiled linens, and cleanup of the facility.

Personal Protective Equipment

Personal protective equipment (PPE) is used to create a barrier between employees and blood or bodily fluids. **Barrier precautions**, such as the use of gloves, are used to minimize the risk of exposure to blood and body fluids. PPE is designed to protect the skin (whether intact or non-intact) and the mucous membranes. Appropriate personal protective equipment should be used by health care workers to protect themselves from exposure to disease-causing

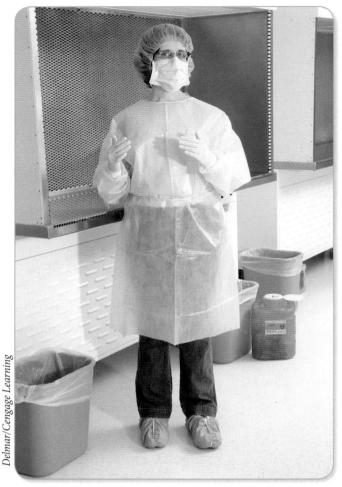

Delmar/Cengage Learning

Figure 1-2 Proper personal protective equipment must be worn when dealing with chemicals or potentially infectious materials.

microorganisms. Personal protective equipment includes gloves, gowns, laboratory coats, face shields, goggles, and masks (see Figure 1-2).

Face shields, goggles, and masks are specifically designed to protect against splashing or splattering of blood, bodily fluids, or any chemical substances. Gowns, laboratory coats, or scrubs should be left at the work site in a special storage area after use. Eye wash stations, which are required by law, should be available in all facilities for emergencies. Employees must be able to flush out their eyes or mucous membranes with water as soon as possible after on-the-job exposure to blood or chemical substances.

In the pharmacy, eye wash stations must be available for flushing contaminants from the eyes (Figure 1-3). Eye wash stations are designed to allow the rinsing of the eyes for a minimum of 15 minutes after contact with a potentially harmful substance. Prior to eye washing, contact lenses should be removed, and the injured person should not rub his or her eyes in order to avoid further absorption of the substance. The injured person should be taken to the emergency department of the local hospital after the eye-washing procedure has been completed.

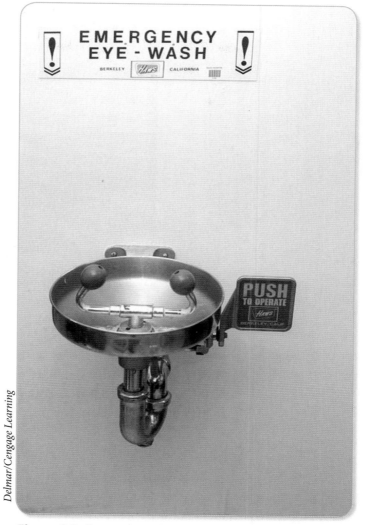

Figure 1-3 Eye wash stations must be available at all facilities.

Housekeeping

OSHA requires that all working surfaces be clean and dry, and free from hazards that may cause tripping or falls. Floors where wet products are used (such as clean rooms) must have drains. Waste receptacles must be leak-proof with tight-fitting covers. A pest extermination service must be employed to ascertain that the workplace is free from insects and other pests. Potable water must be provided for drinking or cleaning. Non-potable water must be provided for industrial use or fire fighting. Restrooms must be provided so that there is at least one toilet for every fifteen employees.

The work area must be cleaned and maintained at all times. The cleaning should be done in compliance with the facilities exposure control plan. Work surfaces and equipment must be appropriately decontaminated. Sharps should be contained in puncture-proof containers (Figure 1-4). Soiled linens and laundry should be handled by the facility and bagged appropriately for disposal or clean up.

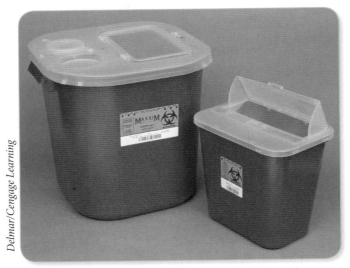

Delmar/Cengage Learning

Figure 1-4 Sharps containers must be used to dispose of needles or broken glass.

HBV Vaccine

Any employee at risk of exposure to blood, body fluids, or other potentially infectious materials must be given the option to have the hepatitis B vaccination at no charge. Refusal of the employee to get the vaccine must be documented. This employee can reconsider getting the vaccine at any time.

Engineering and Work Practice Controls

Engineering controls are defined by OSHA as devices that isolate or remove the bloodborne pathogen hazard from the workplace. These devices such as needleless systems, eye wash stations, hand-washing facilities, and biohazard labels are important factors that can reduce the risk of exposure to microorganisms.

Work practice controls also serve to reduce or eliminate exposure to bloodborne pathogens but also provide infection control. These types of controls consist of hand hygiene procedures, use of PPE, sanitization and disinfection procedures, and procedures for properly handling spills of contaminated waste.

Disposal of Biohazardous Waste

Alert!

Containers for contaminated sharps should be readily accessible to personnel and maintained in an upright position.

Hazardous waste may consist of used needles, or linens and clothing contaminated with blood or body fluids. These items must be properly contained to avoid the risk of exposure to anyone coming into contact with them. Sharps such as glass slides, needles, disposable syringes, or scalpel blades may be placed in leak-proof and puncture-proof containers. Gloves, dressings, paper towels, and other soft hazardous materials must be bagged in leak-proof bags marked with the biohazard symbol (Figure 1-5). If a potentially infectious substance should leak from a bag, the item should be double-bagged before disposal.

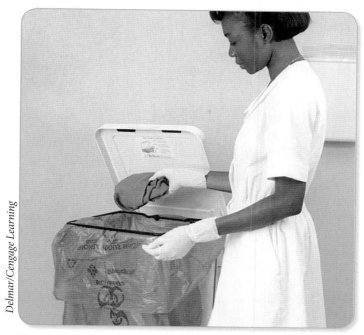

Delmar/Cengage Learning

Figure 1-5 Soiled linens or garments should be disposed of in red plastic biohazard bags.

Training and Documentation

Training is to be given to all employees upon hire. If any aspect of the job changes, additional training should be provided. Training should explain the exposure control plan and what actions need to be followed in the event of an accidental exposure. All training provided as well as a log of employee participation must be documented and maintained on file.

Post-Exposure Follow-up

If an employee is exposed to bloodborne pathogens, the employer is required to provide assistance and support to that employee. A medical evaluation and testing of the employee's blood should be provided at no cost to the employee, the circumstances of the exposure must be documented, the results of the blood tests must be provided to the employee as soon as possible, and post-exposure prophylaxis as well as counseling must be provided by the employer. All communication and documentation of the incident should maintain the confidentiality of the employee. If the employee refuses treatment, there must be documentation of that refusal.

Fire Safety and Emergency Plan

Fire and safety plans must comply with OSHA standards and include written procedures. Most fire safety plans include the use of smoke detectors; fire alarms and pull boxes; fire doors and escapes; and sprinkler systems. Training, including the correct operation of fire extinguishers and other equipment, must be provided by the employer. Fire stairway exits and fire extinguisher locations must be clearly displayed (Figure 1-6).

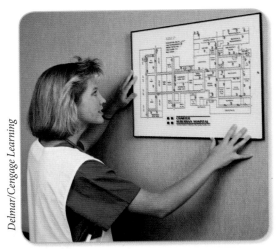

Delmar/Cengage Learning

Figure 1-6 All pharmacy personnel must know emergency evacuation routes in the event of a fire.

Smoke detectors should be located throughout the facility, and installed properly so that they trigger automatic fire alarms when smoke is detected. Fire alarms should have loud horns that sound continuously, and may have a blinking sign that reads "FIRE" as well. They should be mounted on upper walls. Fire alarm pull boxes should be easily activated by pulling down on their handles—they should be mounted on walls so that they are easily reached by most adults.

Overhead fire sprinklers should be mounted on ceilings throughout the facility. They are triggered by the heat levels given off by a fire. Fire stairway exits should have illuminated, ceiling-mounted "EXIT" signs above them, with fire exit stairwells located at each elevator lobby and at the end of each main corridor. Elevators should never be used during a fire.

Emergency procedures should be practiced so that the entire staff knows what to do should a fire or other emergency arise. It is essential that escape routes, as well as the location of fire equipment, be memorized. Fire drills should be conducted periodically so that staff can practice leaving the facility. Conducting these on a periodic basis is important so that new employees will receive the same training as those who have been employed for a longer time.

Fire drills commonly include: checking exits, choosing evacuation routes, verifying that each staff member (as well as customers and other people) leaves the facility in an orderly manner (the use of the daily work schedule helps to confirm that no one may still be inside), rehearsing how to correctly report a fire, practicing the containment of fires by closing off all doors, and when to return to the facility after the "all clear" is given.

Common fire hazards in the workplace may include the following:

- Electrical wires, overloaded circuits, and improperly grounded plugs
- Papers, rags, matches, lighters, and other potentially hazardous items

- Improper protection during oxygen use.

- Smoking where oxygen is used, or elsewhere in the facility.

Fire Prevention

Every workplace has its own policies and procedures concerning fire prevention. Fire occurs with the interaction of three elements (Figure 1-7):

- Source of ignition (also known as the "fuel" for a fire)

- Oxygen (to support the fire)

- Sufficient heat to ignite the fire

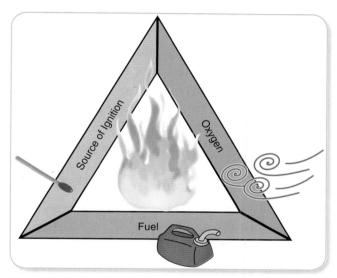

Figure 1-7 The fire triangle displays the elements needed to start a fire.

When a staff member discovers a fire before the fire alarm has sounded, they should make an attempt to extinguish it. If this cannot be done, they should sound the fire alarm and alert the other staff members. The narcotics safe should be checked to make sure that it is locked. All staff should exit the facility, closing doors behind them.

Other procedures that are aimed at preventing or reducing the risk of fire include:

- Posting emergency phone numbers by all telephones.

- Keeping open spaces and hallways clear of clutter.

- Emptying wastepaper cans into proper receptacles.

- Using proper electrical cords to handle large power loads, with three-prong grounded plugs.

- Reporting identified electrical hazards.

- Reporting smoke or burning smells.

- Not stacking linen and supplies closer than 18 inches to the ceiling so that the fire sprinkler system will be effective during a fire.

The four types of fire extinguishers that are commonly used are as follows:

- Carbon dioxide (Type B and C)
- Water (Type A)
- Multipurpose dry chemical (Type A, B, and C)
- Regular dry chemical (Type B and C)

Electrical Safety

Electricity can be a major physical hazard. All electrical equipment must be properly grounded by following the manufacturer's instructions and local electrical codes. Instruments must be disconnected from their power supply before any work on them is started. This includes minor repairs such as replacing light bulbs inside equipment such as microscopes or drying ovens. All electrical cords and plugs must be kept in good repair. There should be no exposed wires or frayed cords. Circuits must not be overloaded, because overloading creates a fire hazard and can cause equipment damage. Extension cords should only be used in an emergency because they can create electrical safety hazards as well as cause an employee to trip.

Environmental Pollution

OSHA requires that workplaces have clean air provided by an exhaust ventilation system. These systems remove contaminated air and return clean, filtered air. Effective air filtration involves the removing of approximately 90 percent of all particles found in the airflow stream.

Noise pollution is defined as levels of noise that are uncomfortable. Noise pollution often occurs in the workplace due to visitor traffic, employees, and pharmacy equipment. It can result in hearing loss, overload of auditory stimuli, and disorganization. Sensory overload can increase anxiety and other conditions that are not conducive to a healthy working environment. Quiet sound levels should be maintained, even by the use of earplugs if applicable.

Latex Allergy

Latex products are made from a rubber obtained from trees found in Brazil. Certain people may experience an allergic response to the proteins contained in the milky fluid used to manufacture latex products (such as rubber gloves used in the laboratory) as well as the chemical added during their manufacture. The three types of allergic reactions to latex are as follows:

1. allergic contact dermatitis (the most common type).
2. irritant contact dermatitis, and
3. immediate hypersensitivity (a systemic reaction).

In 1992, OSHA issued regulations requiring health care workers to wear gloves and other protective devices to safeguard against bloodborne pathogens. As a result, many people were placed at risk for developing latex

Alert!

Fires can be kept from spreading via the use of doors that close automatically when a fire alarm sounds, automatic sprinkler systems, smoke detectors, and fire exits.

allergy, with latex being present not only in gloves, but in blood pressure cuffs, stethoscopes, catheters, wound drains, and many other pieces of equipment. Studies have shown that about 8 to 12 percent of regularly exposed health care workers are sensitive to latex (NIOSH, 1997).

It is recommended that if latex gloves are worn, they should be powder-free and low-allergen. These gloves are less likely than powdered ones to produce allergic responses (Ferrie, 2004).

Work-Related Musculoskeletal Disorders

About one-third of all occupational injuries reported by employers are work-related musculoskeletal disorders. OSHA has issued mandatory standards requiring all employers to set up **ergonomic** programs to prevent such injuries. The word *ergonomic* means "adapting the environment and using techniques and equipment to prevent injury to the body." Ergonomic standards state that a 51-pound stable object with handles is the heaviest amount of weight that can be safely lifted. Employers must provide all of the following information to their employees:

- common musculoskeletal disorders and hazards;
- how to report musculoskeletal signs and symptoms;
- signs and symptoms of musculoskeletal disorders;
- the importance of reporting these disorders early; and
- a summary of the requirement of OSHA standards.

The eight commandments for lifting to decrease the risk of injury to the body include:

1. Plan your lift and test the load (Figure 1-8A);
2. Ask for help (Figure 1-8B).
3. Get a firm footing (Figure 1-8C).
4. Bend your knees (Figure 1-8D).
5. Tighten your abdominal muscles (Figure 1-8E).
6. Lift with your legs (Figure 1-8F).
7. Keep the load close (Figure 1-8G).
8. Keep your back upright (Figure 1-8H).

Exposure Reduction to Chemotherapeutic Agents

Pharmacy technicians must be very careful to avoid exposure to radiopharmaceutical substances. Radiation exposure can negatively affect the tissues of the body. Radiation exposure can be reduced by:

- Increasing the distance between personnel and radiation sources.
- Decreasing the amount of time personnel are in contact with radiation sources.

Alert!

If you experience signs of an allergy when wearing latex gloves, ask your pharmacist for latex-free or hypoallergenic gloves made of nitrile or vinyl.

Alert!

The back support belt works by keeping your spine in good alignment. Do not lift more than you would if you were not wearing the belt. Using a back support belt does not make you stronger.

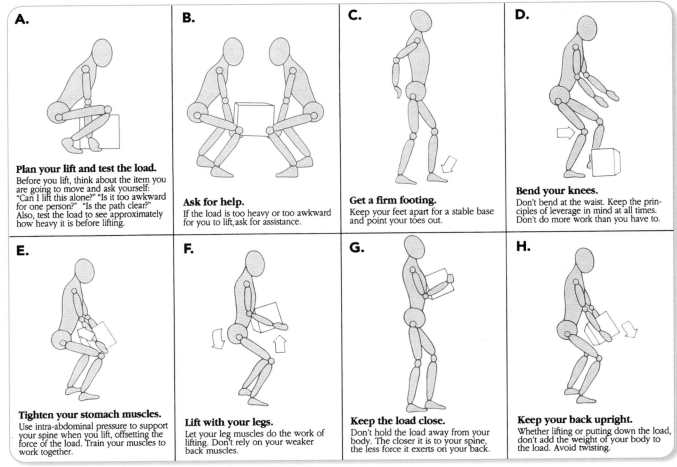

A.

Plan your lift and test the load.
Before you lift, think about the item you are going to move and ask yourself: "Can I lift this alone?" "Is it too awkward for one person?" "Is the path clear?" Also, test the load to see approximately how heavy it is before lifting.

B.

Ask for help.
If the load is too heavy or too awkward for you to lift, ask for assistance.

C.

Get a firm footing.
Keep your feet apart for a stable base and point your toes out.

D.

Bend your knees.
Don't bend at the waist. Keep the principles of leverage in mind at all times. Don't do more work than you have to.

E.

Tighten your stomach muscles.
Use intra-abdominal pressure to support your spine when you lift, offsetting the force of the load. Train your muscles to work together.

F.

Lift with your legs.
Let your leg muscles do the work of lifting. Don't rely on your weaker back muscles.

G.

Keep the load close.
Don't hold the load away from your body. The closer it is to your spine, the less force it exerts on your back.

H.

Keep your back upright.
Whether lifting or putting down the load, don't add the weight of your body to the load. Avoid twisting.

Figure 1-8 Eight rules for lifting and moving. (Reprinted with permission from Ergodyne Corporation, St. Paul, MN)

- Monitoring radiation exposure with film badges (Figure 1-9).
- Labeling all potentially radioactive materials.
- Using appropriate radiation shields.

Ergonomics

Ergonomics serves to enhance workplace design to improve productivity as well as reduce fatigue and discomfort. A properly designed workplace reduces employee injury on the job. Employers must provide employees basic information about what types of workplace injuries can occur, the signs and symptoms of those injuries, how to report an injury, and an overview of OSHA's ergonomics standard.

Workplace Violence

Employees in the medical field have an increased risk of injury due to violence in the workplace. The majority of violence in the workplace comes from assault. Employers are encouraged to develop and maintain violence

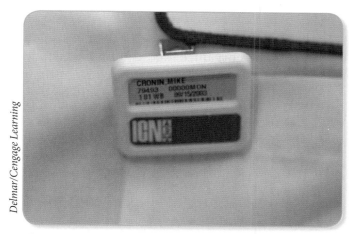

Delmar/Cengage Learning

Figure 1-9 Radiation monitoring device.

prevention programs. The employer's approach should exemplify a balanced concern for the welfare of the employees as well as that of clients. Employees should be involved and engaged in the prevention programs. Engineering controls can be implemented to foster a safer work environment, such as the use of security cameras and alarm systems, construction of safe areas or barriers, and having adequate exits. Administrative and work practice controls to minimize risk of violence in the workplace consist of educating and training employees, stating expectations of clients, establishing rapport with security or law enforcement officers, and maintaining adequate staff coverage, as well as implementing policies for dealing with aggressive or agitated clients.

STANDARDS AND REGULATIONS WITHIN THE FIELD OF PHARMACY

State boards of pharmacy implement standards and regulations for the industry within their states. These rules are more specific to the industry than many of the more general OSHA standards and regulations that are either specific to the medical industry as a whole or the broader workforce in the United States as a whole. Individual facilities may also have particular standards and rules their employees are expected to know, understand, and uphold. Pharmacy technicians must always follow the policies and procedures for storing, compounding, preparing, and dispensing medications. They must be familiar with the rules and regulations of their board of pharmacy as well as those of OSHA.

Storing Medication Safely

Medication should always be stored by carefully following the manufacturer's specifications. Most drugs are stored at room temperature, though many must be kept refrigerated—each drug label or packaging should be checked to determine the correct storage procedure. Most retail pharmacies store their medications alphabetically by brand name. Some organize medications alphabetically by generic name, placing all different manufacturers' versions of the same generic drug together in one group. There should be enough space allowed between medications so that the chance of accidentally choosing the wrong one is minimized.

Safety requires that chemical substances should be separated from actual medications. Acids and cleaning supplies such as bleach must be stored separately, away from medications. Each board of pharmacy has special regulations for the safe storage of potentially hazardous substances, especially cytotoxic and radioactive substances. These substances should be stored in their own areas, away from other types of substances.

Pharmacy Storage Equipment

Drug storage areas should be properly ventilated. Shelving should be strong enough to support all of the medications. There should be adequate light to easily read the labels of the medications. Airflow around the medications should not be restricted. Labeling adhered to shelving that indicates the correct location of each drug should be consistent with the information about each drug that is stored in the computer system. Proper location labeling makes it easier and quicker to access a specific drug from the pharmacy shelving.

Safely Preparing Medications

The occurrence of errors can be reduced by limiting the amount of medications stored, as well as limiting volumes and number of concentrations of each medication. Safely preparing medications is essential in preventing medication errors that could harm a patient. When a pharmacy technician prepares, compounds, or dispenses medications, care must be taken to avoid any errors. Contamination with microorganisms may occur during preparation. Therefore, hand washing and clean technique are critical. During compounding, injury or harm to the technician or coworkers must be prevented. Employees should observe OSHA regulations concerning needle sticks and injury with other sharps during sterile compounding. Likewise, care should be taken with medication bags and all other equipment in order to avoid spills, contamination, and transfer of bloodborne pathogens.

Clean Work Environment

A clean work environment is essential for compounding. In general, equipment and instruments need to be cleaned immediately after each use. Visible residue must first be removed, followed by disinfection and sterilization. Sanitization decreases amounts of microorganisms

Alert!

The following factors may result in unsafe scenarios during the preparation of medications: drug errors, strength errors, wrong dosage forms, and incorrect or incomplete label instructions.

to safe levels, and removes blood and other body fluids that may carry pathogens. The overall cleaning of the workplace includes regular dusting and vacuuming, as well as prompt changing of air conditioning filters. Chemical disinfectants are used to clean work surfaces, heat-sensitive equipment, rubberized equipment, various appliances, floor mats, sinks, and cabinets.

Safe Handling of Cytotoxic and Hazardous Medications

Cytotoxic medications are those that may cause cancer, mutations, or harm to a developing embryo or fetus. They may also cause damage to skin, mucous membranes, and eyes, leading to ulcerations and tissue death.

When cytotoxic or hazardous drugs are prepared and compounded, there is a high potential for skin contact, splashing, and inhalation of toxic elements. Safe handling is essential during the activities of withdrawal of medications from vials, opening of ampoules, and expelling air from a syringe when measuring medications.

Cytotoxic medications should be prepared within a vertical laminar airflow hood in order to minimize exposure to the person preparing them. Proper protective equipment for cytotoxic medications includes non-powdered latex or hypoallergenic gloves, and a disposable gown with elastic or knit cuffs. Vials should be vented prior to use in order to reduce internal pressure. External surfaces that may have been splashed with a cytotoxic medication should be wiped down with alcohol pads. Ampoules should be snapped open only by holding an alcohol pad over the breakage point. Hands should be washed after glove removal and between glove changes.

Proper handling and disposal of cytotoxic and hazardous medications is essential in reducing potential exposures, following disposal guidelines set forth by local, state, and federal agencies. Radiation safety standards are established by the state boards of pharmacy. These include limits for radiation doses, levels of radiation in an area, and concentrations of radioactivity in the air and waste water. Limits also exist for the amount of radioactivity in disposed waste. Precautionary procedures are enforced by the U.S. Nuclear Regulatory Commission (***http://www.nrc.gov***). Many other aspects of health and safety are also important, but radiation protection is the most regulated area.

In case of contact with cytotoxic medications, the affected area should be thoroughly washed with soap and water. A scrub brush should not be used so that the skin stays intact. Eyes should be immediately flushed with water for at least 15 minutes. The person who has been exposed to cytotoxic medications must then be taken to the emergency department. In nuclear pharmacy practice, health and safety are crucial elements.

Cleaning Up a Spill

Pharmacies have spill cleanup kits in areas where potentially harmful chemicals and substances are used (see Figure 1-10). Most spills should be cleaned up by using these kits, and not by ordinary paper towels. Absorbents and neutralizers in these kits are designed to clean up specific acids, alkalis, and other substances. If a biohazard such as blood is spilled, bleach is recommended for the cleanup in order to kill the pathogens that may be carried. If an extremely toxic substance is spilled, it is advisable that a specially trained hazardous cleanup team be called in.

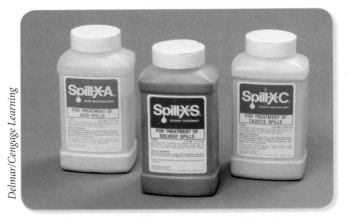

Delmar/Cengage Learning

Figure 1-10 Absorbent substances used to clean hazardous chemical spills.

For hazardous material spills, the following steps should be followed:

- Put on gloves and other personal protective equipment.

- Bring appropriate supplies and a hazardous waste container to where the spill has occurred.

- Pick up broken glass with tongs or other equipment—never use your hands.

- Dispose of broken glass properly.

- Wipe up the spill with appropriate materials as found in the spill kit and as regulated by the policies and procedures manual.

- Dispose of these cleaning materials in a biohazard container.

- After completing a thorough cleaning of the area, disinfect with an approved disinfectant.

- Remove gloves and properly discard.

- Wash your hands thoroughly.

Hazardous Waste Management

Hazardous wastes should be disposed of only by using a licensed disposal service or facility. Most hazardous wastes are disposed of in designated landfills, surface impoundments (such as designated pits, ponds, or lagoons), waste piles, land treatment units, or injection wells. Proper management of hazardous wastes includes regulation on air emissions, closure of containers, proper cleanup, monitoring of ground water, restrictions on land disposal, and strict permits.

Defining Hazardous Waste

Any waste that may be potentially dangerous or harmful to human health or the environment should be considered **hazardous waste**. A hazardous waste may be ignitable, corrosive, reactive, or toxic. These wastes may be either liquids, solids, gases, or sludges. The EPA defines hazardous waste by placing each type of waste into one of three categories: the *F-list* (non-specific source wastes), the *K-list* (source-specific wastes), and the *P-list or U-list* (discarded commercial chemicals). Ignitable wastes are those that can create fires under certain conditions. Corrosive wastes are those that can corrode various types of metal containers. Reactive wastes are unstable, and may cause explosions, fumes, gases, or vapors. Toxic wastes are harmful or fatal when ingested or otherwise absorbed. Table 1-2 shows the EPA designations of hazardous wastes.

TABLE 1-2   EPA Hazardous Waste Designations

Designation	Type of Waste	Industry
F-List	Non-specific source wastes (solvents, sludges, plating solutions and residues, reactants, etc.)	Various—from common manufacturing and industrial processes
K-List	Source-specific wastes (various types of sludges, oven residue, distillation byproducts, bottom tars, process residues, adsorbents, etc.)	Specific industries such as petroleum refining, pesticide manufacturing, etc.
P-List or U-List	Discarded and unused commercial chemicals (acetone, aluminum phosphide, arsenic oxide, benzene, creosote, epinephrine, ethanol, fluorine, mercury fulminate, nitric oxide, nitrogen oxide, etc.)	Various

Disposal of Hazardous Wastes

Biohazard symbols should be displayed on specific waste container to ensure that all employees are aware of the contents (Figure 1-11). A health care facilities must have guidelines for hazardous materials per th OSHA Act of 1991. When disposing of hazardous materials, the pharmac technician should always:

- Wear gloves.

- Use proper containers.

- Ensure that all waste is properly labeled.

- Use care to avoid punctures and tearing.

- Disinfect carts used to carry waste materials.

- Dispose of waste in designated areas only.

- Wash hands after disposing of hazardous materials.

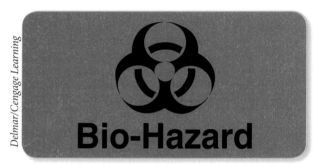

Figure 1-11 Biohazard symbols alert the pharmacy technician to hazardous materials.

Companies that specialize in removal and disposal of hazardous waste are usually used by medical facilities, and therefore, cleaning staff should no empty hazardous waste containers. When hazardous waste bags are change by health care workers, the worker must wear gloves, masks, and protectiv eyewear. These bags should be placed inside a second hazardous waste bag i there is any chance of leakage.

Disposal of drugs by flushing them down sinks or toilets is becoming increasingly regulated. Many drugs can pollute water supplies, and the dangers of disposing of them via these methods are becoming more focuse on every day. Many unexpected drugs have been found in public wate sources, including acetaminophen, erythromycin, fluoxetine, and albuterol Contaminants have caused mutations in fish and other water life.

As of 2007, it is now advised that expired prescription drugs be removed from their original containers and mixed with coffee grounds o cat litter, then placed in empty cans or sealed bags and thrown in the trash. I possible, it is advised that prescription drugs be turned in to pharmaceutica "take-back" locations. A list of these locations across the United States can be found at: ***http://www.teleosis.org/*** (Click on "Green Pharmacy" and then "Medicine Take Back Locations".)

Drugs that may still be flushed include the following: fentanyl and fentanyl citrate, methylphenidate, oxycodone and oxycodone/acetaminophen, morphine sulfate, entecavir, atazanavir sulfate, gatifloxacin, stavudine, meperidine hydrochloride, and sodium oxybate.

The policies and procedures concerning hazardous waste disposal and management may differ widely between facilities, areas of government with jurisdiction, the EPA, and OSHA. Special attention must be given to the disposal of chemotherapy agents, AIDS medications, certain infusion therapies, all cytotoxic agents, and all radioactive agents. Anyone involved in home infusion must comply strictly with government and other regulations concerning disposal, and their actions are strictly controlled by home infusion regulatory agencies.

Summary

The Occupational Health and Safety Administration (OSHA) is responsible for workplace safety rules and their enforcement. OSHA strives to protect health care employees from biological and chemical hazards by requiring written exposure control plans to be used concerning protective measures against bloodborne pathogen transmission. Records of potentially hazardous chemicals in the workplace must be kept by employers, and these chemicals must be labeled and sealed correctly. Employers must provide training about OSHA regulations, fire safety, and hazard communication. Personal protective equipment should always be worn if there is a danger of possible injury or contamination.

Special training about OSHA should be provided initially as an employee begins working at the workplace, and then annually if new procedures are developed. Fire extinguishers and fire alarm pull boxes must be located throughout the workplace. Every health care worker should know and practice fire and evacuation plans.

Hazards in the workplace must be minimized and employees should know and understand how to protect themselves from all potential hazards and hazardous materials. Proper infection-control principles can reduce the transmission of microorganisms. Medications should always be safely stored, and the occurrence of medication errors can be reduced by safe medication preparation procedures. Cytotoxic and hazardous medications must be handled with extreme care during preparation and compounding. It is important that all hazardous wastes be disposed of by licensed disposal companies.

Related Internet Sites

http://www.pharmacy.ohio-state.edu (Click on "Research"; click on "Safety Information"; then click on "List of Hazardous Substances.")

http://www.osha.gov (Click on "O" in the A-Z Index; click on "OSHA Technical Manual - (OTM)"; scroll down to "Section vi: Health-Care Facilities"; Click on "Chapter 2. Controlling Occupational Exposure to Hazardous Drugs.")

http://www.uth.tmc.edu

http://www.utmb.edu

http://www.osha.gov (Click on "O" in the A-Z Index; click on "OSHA Regulations – (29 CFR)"; click on "PART 1910 Occupational Safety and Health Standards"; scroll down to and click on "1910.94 - Ventilation.")

http://dohs.ors.od.nih.gov (Click on "Publications and Policies"; scroll down to and click on "Recommendations for the Safe Use of Handling of Cytotoxic Drugs, NIH Publication No. 92-2621.")

www.epa.gov/osw/hazard/index.htm

http://www.drugtopics.com

REVIEW QUESTIONS

Multiple Choice

1. Standard Precautions are issued by:

    A. Centers for Disease Control and Prevention
    B. Food and Drug Administration
    C. Health and Human Services
    D. Occupational Safety and Health Administration

2. Pharmacy technicians that deal with radiopharmaceutical substances can reduce radiation exposure by which of the following methods?

    A. monitoring radiation exposure with film badges
    B. maximizing time in contact with radiation sources
    C. labeling all radiation exposure sites in their body
    D. using appropriate gowns

3. The Bloodborne Pathogen Standard is primarily concerned with:

    A. reducing the transmission of HBV, HCV, and HIV infections
    B. protecting the employer from lawsuits
    C. regulating the use of personal protective equipment
    D. taking blood samples from patients

4. The exposure control plan must be reviewed every:

    A. 5 years   C. 2 years
    B. 3 years   D. year

5. Hazardous wastes should only be disposed of by using which of the following?

    A. burning them in an approved container
    B. flushing them down a toilet
    C. using a licensed disposal service or facility
    D. throwing them into the facility's trash containers

6. According to ergonomic standards, which of the following is the heaviest amount of weight that can be safely lifted?

    A. 25 lbs   C. 51 lbs
    B. 42 lbs   D. 62 lbs

7. All of the following are potential fire hazards, except:

    A. overloaded circuits
    B. plugs that are improperly grounded

    C. insufficient heat to ignite a fire

    D. frayed electrical wires

8. Appropriate personal protective equipment should be used by pharmacy technicians to protect from exposure to:

    A. fire

    B. carbon dioxide

    C. pathogen

    D. all of the above

9. OSHA standards require which of the following?

    A. a written schedule for cleaning

    B. cleaning only when needed

    C. cleaning only after procedures

    D. cleaning by the cleaning staff only

10. The four types of fire extinguishers that are commonly used include all of the following, except:

    A. regular dry chemical (Type B and C)

    B. water (Type A)

    C. multipurpose dry chemical (Type A, B, and C)

    D. carbon monoxide (Type B and C)

11. If a pharmacy technician is sensitive to latex gloves, he or she:

    A. should ask for non-latex gloves

    B. should put powder in the gloves

    C. should wear the latex gloves anyway

    D. need not wear gloves

12. Fire occurs with the interaction of three elements. Which of the following is not one of these elements?

    A. carbon monoxide

    B. oxygen

    C. an ignition source

    D. sufficient heat to ignite the fir

Fill in the Blank

1. Employees are required to abide by all of the safety and health standards that apply to their _____.

2. Fire safety plans must comply with _____ standards.

3. In the event of a fire, you must follow your workplace's _____ and _____ manual for fire containment and evacuation.

4. Any electrical shocks should be _____.

5. Radiation exposure can affect targeted or _____ tissues of patients and pharmacy technicians.

6. Employers who have more than _____ employees must maintain work-related injury and illness records.

7. Pharmacy technicians who prepare or compound chemotherapeutic agents are exposed to _____ hazards.

8. OSHA is part of the Department of _____.

9. The ability of a microorganism to produce disease is known as _____.

10. Sharps such as glass slides and disposable syringes may be placed in _____ containers.

LAB: USE OF THE MSDS SHEET

Objective

To locate information on hazardous products in the workplace and to properly use that information.

Equipment

Hazardous Communication Plan
MSDS sheets
Pen and paper

Directions

At your clinical site or in your school's lab, locate the hazard communication plan. Review the list of hazardous substances that can be found in the facility. Identify a product from the list and look up the MSDS form for that product. List the possible hazards that the product poses, outline the handling and storage of that product, identify the exposure control protection that should be used, and list the actions that should be taken if an accidental exposure occurs.

REFERENCES

DeLaune, S. C., & Ladner, P. K. (2006). *Fundamentals of Nursing: Standards and Practice*. Clifton Park, NY: Delmar Cengage Learning.

Hegner, B. R., Acello, B., & Caldwell, E. (2008). *Nursing Assistant: A Nursing Process Approach*. Clifton Park, NY: Delmar Cengage Learning.

NIOSH. (1997). *Musculoskeletal Disorders and Workplace Factors*. Cincinnati, OH: National Technical Information Service.

Prescriptions and Drug Classifications

OBJECTIVES

Upon completion of this chapter, the student should be able to:

1. Define what is meant by over-the-counter drugs.
2. Describe drug standards and references.
3. Identify drug classifications.
4. Discuss proper drug disposal.
5. Explain the principal drug actions.
6. Discuss drug routes of administration.
7. Identify drug forms.
8. Describe storage and handling of drugs.

GLOSSARY

Anaphylaxis – An acute, severe, systemic hypersensitivity allergic reaction.

Expiration dates – Estimated dates at which drugs are no longer at their effective potential; they are based on proper storage in approved containers away from such factors as heat and humidity.

Legend drug – Another name for a prescription drug.

Medication administration record (MAR) – Documentation of the drug ordered, when it was given, how it was administered, the dosage given, and who gave it; used within the hospital setting.

Over-the-counter (OTC) – Medications that are deemed safe for use without the oversight of a physician.

Parenteral – Administration route other than through the digestive tract; most commonly refers to drugs administered intravenously.

Potentiation – Undesirable or desirable increasing or diminishing of another drug's actions.

Physician's Desk Reference (PDR) – The standard medication reference book found in most medical offices; it lists most available medications.

Physician's order form – Documentation used in the hospital setting to order medications for a patient.

Prescription – A physician's order for the preparation and administration of a drug or device for a patient.

OUTLINE

United States Pharmacopoeia/ National Formulary – A list of drugs for which standards have been established by the government; it is recognized as the official list of drug standards, as enforced by the FDA.

Vasoconstrictor – Any substance that causes narrowing of the blood vessels.

OVERVIEW

Pharmacy technicians use drug knowledge and individual patient information to maximize the therapeutic effects (and minimize the adverse effects) of various drugs. Technicians must be familiar with the structure of prescriptions and principles of drug actions. When preparing drugs, the technician is required to be familiar with prescription and nonprescription drugs, drug references, drug classifications, drug routes, and different drug forms.

PRESCRIPTION DRUGS

The process of writing a **prescription** requires prescribers to sign each order they write for the dispensing of drugs. State law governs the practice of prescribing medications for patients. All of the Schedule II controlled substances require a prescription for their legal use, as well as certain other drugs (including the cardiac drug *digoxin* and the **vasoconstrictor** *epinephrine*). Prescription drugs are also called **legend drugs.** A prescription is a legal document and has specific elements that must be present (Figure 2-1). The pharmacy technician must be knowledgeable about the parts of a prescription and what makes a prescription legal.

Parts of a Prescription

1. The physician's name, address, telephone number, and registration number.
2. The patient's name, address, and the date on which the prescription is written.
3. The *superscription* that includes the symbol Rx ("take thou").
4. The *inscription* that states the names and quantities of ingredients to be included in the medication.
5. The *subscription* that gives directions to the pharmacist for filling the prescription.
6. The *signature* (Sig) that gives the directions for the patient.
7. The physician's signature blanks. Where signed, indicates if a generic substitute is allowed or if the medication is to be dispensed as written.
8. This is where the physician indicates whether or not the prescription can be refilled.
9. Direction to the pharmacist to label the medication appropriately.

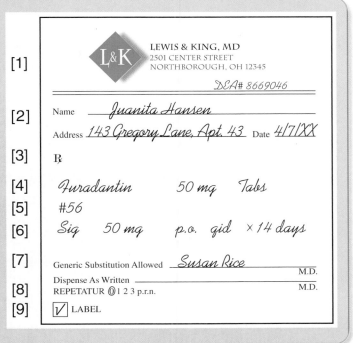

Figure 2-1 Prescriptions are written legal documents that must contain specific elements.

Hospitals have special forms used for recording drug orders, usuall[y] called a **physician's order form**. Pharmacy technicians should be familia[r] with these forms as well. Prescriptions and medication orders are ofte[n] handwritten, so the pharmacy technician must be able to interpret th[e] handwriting of the physician or other health care professional who filled ou[t] the form. If there is any doubt, seek confirmation of what is being requeste[d.] Figure 2-2 shows a sample physician's order form.

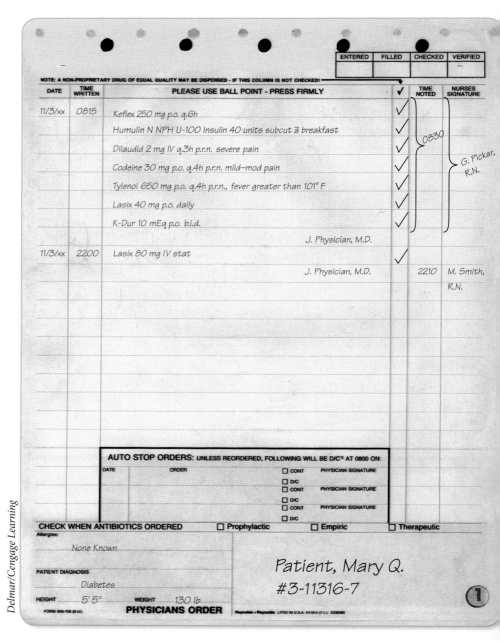

		ENTERED	FILLED	CHECKED	VERIFIED

NOTE: A NON-PROPRIETARY DRUG OF EQUAL QUALITY MAY BE DISPENSED - IF THIS COLUMN IS NOT CHECKED!

DATE	TIME WRITTEN	PLEASE USE BALL POINT - PRESS FIRMLY	✓	TIME NOTED	NURSES SIGNATURE
11/3/xx	0815	Keflex 250 mg p.o. q.6h	✓		
		Humulin N NPH U-100 Insulin 40 units subcut ā breakfast	✓	0830	
		Dilaudid 2 mg IV q.3h p.r.n. severe pain	✓		G. Pickar, R.N.
		Codeine 30 mg p.o. q.4h p.r.n. mild–mod pain	✓		
		Tylenol 650 mg p.o. q.4h p.r.n., fever greater than 101° F	✓		
		Lasix 40 mg p.o. daily	✓		
		K-Dur 10 mEq p.o. b.i.d.	✓		
		J. Physician, M.D.			
11/3/xx	2200	Lasix 80 mg IV stat	✓		
		J. Physician, M.D.		2210	M. Smith, R.N.

AUTO STOP ORDERS: UNLESS REORDERED, FOLLOWING WILL BE D/C° AT 0800 ON:

DATE	ORDER		
		☐ CONT ☐ D/C	PHYSICIAN SIGNATURE
		☐ CONT ☐ D/C	PHYSICIAN SIGNATURE
		☐ CONT ☐ D/C	PHYSICIAN SIGNATURE

CHECK WHEN ANTIBIOTICS ORDERED ☐ Prophylactic ☐ Empiric ☐ Therapeutic

Allergies:
None Known

PATIENT DIAGNOSIS
Diabetes

HEIGHT 5'5" WEIGHT 130 lb

FORM 959-708 (8-XX) **PHYSICIANS ORDER** Reynolds • Reynolds LITHO IN U.S.A.

Patient, Mary Q.
#3-11316-7

①

Delmar/Cengage Learning

Figure 2-2 Physician's order form.

Drug orders from physician's order forms are also transcribed to a **medication administration record (MAR)**, which is used as a guide to check the drug order, prepare the correct dosage, and record the drug administered and time of administration. Pharmacy technicians should also be familiar with this type of form. Figure 2-3 shows a sample medication administration record.

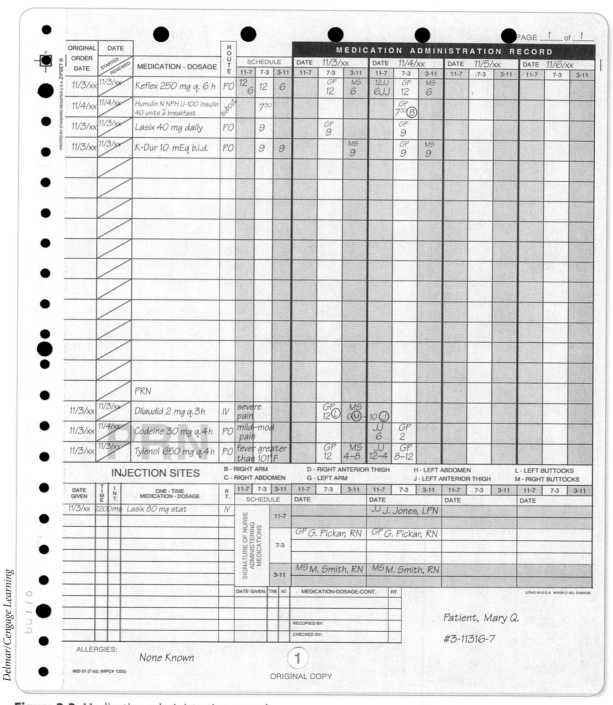

Figure 2-3 Medication administration record.

Exercise: Interpreting Prescriptions

Objective: To practice reading prescriptions and be able to interpret the handwriting of physicians.

Transcribe each of the prescriptions presented or enter them into the computer in your laboratory setting.

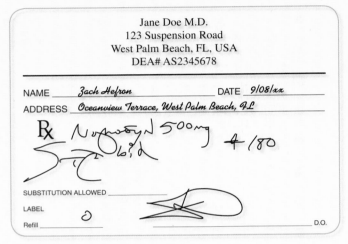

Figure 2-4A Sample prescription.

_____

_____

_____

_____

Terry Jones M.D.
987 Wellness Street
Fort Lauderdale, FL, USA
DEA# AS9876543

NAME _____ Julie Phelps _____ DATE __12/3/xx__
ADDRESS _ 120 Century Dr. Ft. Lauderdale, FL _

℞ Tegretol 200mg #270
tid

SUBSTITUTION ALLOWED _____

LABEL

Refill _____   D.O.

Figure 2-4B Sample prescription.

_____

_____

_____

_____

Exercise: Interpreting Prescriptions (Continued)

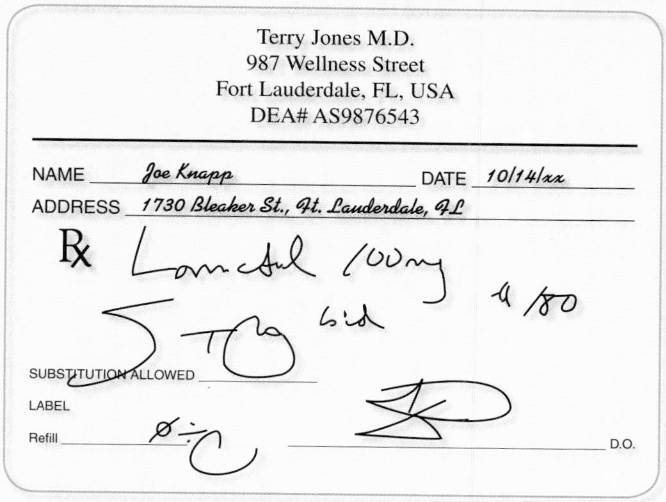

Terry Jones M.D.
987 Wellness Street
Fort Lauderdale, FL, USA
DEA# AS9876543

NAME _Joe Knapp_ DATE _10/14/xx_
ADDRESS _1730 Bleaker St., Ft. Lauderdale, FL_

Rx Lamictal 100mg # 80
     sig bid

SUBSTITUTION ALLOWED _____
LABEL
Refill _____   D.O.

Figure 2-4C Sample prescription.

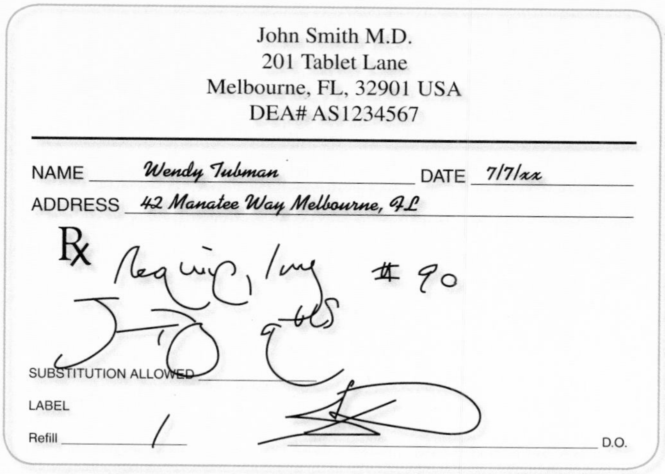

_____
_____
_____
_____

John Smith M.D.
201 Tablet Lane
Melbourne, FL, 32901 USA
DEA# AS1234567

NAME _Wendy Tubman_ DATE _7/7/xx_
ADDRESS _42 Manatee Way Melbourne, FL_

Rx Requip 1mg # 90
     q-6S

SUBSTITUTION ALLOWED _____
LABEL
Refill _____1_____   D.O.

Figure 2-4D Sample prescription.

_____
_____
_____
_____

Exercise: Interpreting Prescriptions (Continued)

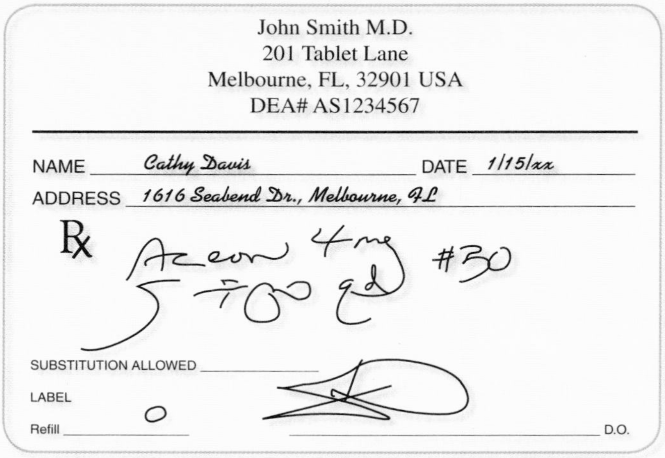
John Smith M.D.
201 Tablet Lane
Melbourne, FL, 32901 USA
DEA# AS1234567

NAME Cathy Davis DATE 1/15/xx
ADDRESS 1616 Seabend Dr., Melbourne, FL

℞ Aceon 4mg #30
Sig i po qd

SUBSTITUTION ALLOWED
LABEL
Refill 0
D.O.

Figure 2-4E Sample prescription.

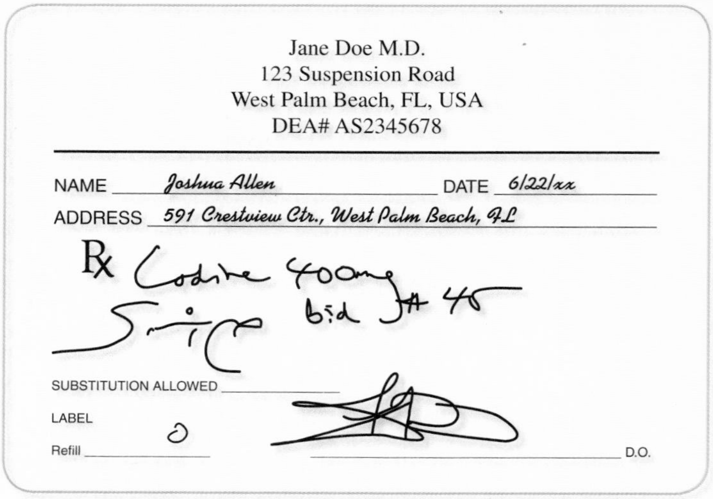
Jane Doe M.D.
123 Suspension Road
West Palm Beach, FL, USA
DEA# AS2345678

NAME Joshua Allen DATE 6/22/xx
ADDRESS 591 Crestview Ctr., West Palm Beach, FL

℞ Codine 400mg
Sig i po bid #45

SUBSTITUTION ALLOWED
LABEL
Refill 0
D.O.

Figure 2-4F Sample prescription.

Exercise: Interpreting Prescriptions (Continued)

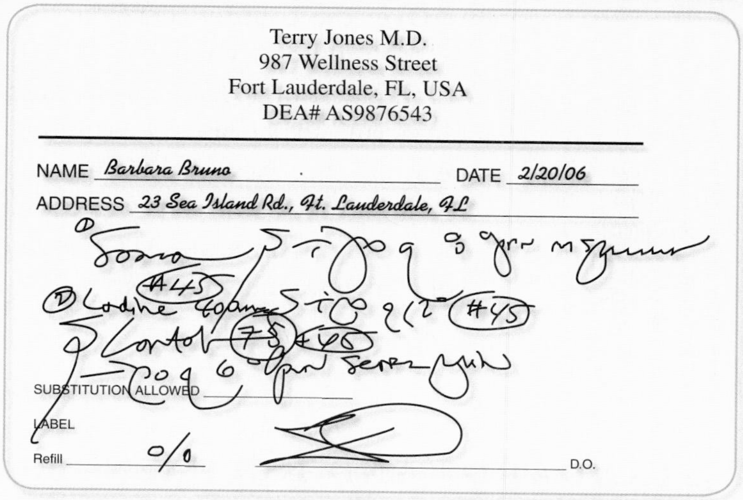

Terry Jones M.D.
987 Wellness Street
Fort Lauderdale, FL, USA
DEA# AS9876543

NAME *Barbara Bruno*   DATE *2/20/06*
ADDRESS *23 Sea Island Rd., Ft. Lauderdale, FL*

SUBSTITUTION ALLOWED

LABEL

Refill _____ 0/0   D.O.

Figure 2-4G Sample prescription.

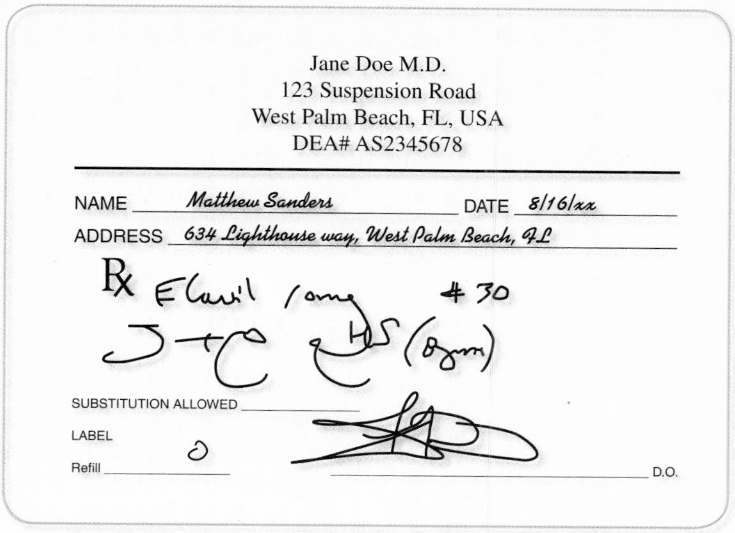

Jane Doe M.D.
123 Suspension Road
West Palm Beach, FL, USA
DEA# AS2345678

NAME *Matthew Sanders*   DATE *8/16/xx*
ADDRESS *634 Lighthouse way, West Palm Beach, FL*

℞ Elavil 10mg   # 30

SUBSTITUTION ALLOWED

LABEL

Refill _____   D.O.

Figure 2-4H Sample prescription.

Note

There are additional examples of handwritten prescriptions for students to practice with at the end of this book in Part II, Self-Evaluation

NONPRESCRIPTION DRUGS

Alert!

Supplements, including vitamins and herbs, are not regulated by the FDA in the same manner as OTC medications. Many herbal supplements interact with legend and OTC drugs. When taking other medications, patients should contact the physician or pharmacist before beginning these supplements.

Over-the-counter (OTC) or nonprescription drugs, are easily accessible by the public at virtually any type of retail store. The Food and Drug Administration (FDA) considers these drugs safe enough to use without a physician's advice or a prescription. Although considered safe, patients must be aware that these drugs can cause harm if not taken exactly as directed, taking into account every caution or warning that is on the medication's packaging. Common OTC products include aspirin, ibuprofen, herbal supplements, and vitamins.

DRUG STANDARDS AND REFERENCES

The **United States Pharmacopoeia/National Formulary** lists drugs for which standards have been established by the government and is recognized as the official list of drug standards as enforced by the FDA. The strength, purity, and quality of drugs are different depending upon their manufacturing processes. This book is updated every 5 years and does not include natural preparations or herbal supplements.

The **Physician's Desk Reference (PDR)** is one of the most widely used reference books found in most offices and clinics. Its seven sections contain in-depth drug information, accompanied by poison control phone numbers, conversion tables, and information about treating drug overdoses. It contains a compilation of drug packet inserts (that would normally be found in the pharmacy on stock bottles), but manufacturers have to pay to have this information listed in the PDR. As a result, the PDR does not contain all medication manufactured in the U.S.

Using the PDR

The pink section of the PDR lists brand names and generic names of drugs. Classifications or categories of drugs are included in the blue section of the book. The white section contains product information, with another white section containing an alphabetical arrangement by drug manufacturer.

If the pharmacy technician knows the brand name of a drug, it can be located in the pink section, which provides information on the manufacturer and other page numbers for more information. If the classification of the drug is known, turn to the blue section to locate its category. All controlled substances are listed in the PDR with the symbol C (to indicate "controlled") followed by a roman numeral, II, III, IV, or V (to indicate its drug schedule).

Exercise

Objective: To become familiar with the information that can be found in the PDR and effectively use it as a tool to look up drug information.

Using a PDR, list the correct drug classification and schedule for each of the following:

Methylphenidate _____

Alprazolam _____

Secobarbital _____

Hydrocodone _____

Diphenoxylate with atropine_____

Other Drug References

There are other drug reference sources available besides the USP and the PDR. The book titled *Drug Facts and Comparisons* is more comprehensive and is more widely used in pharmacies. It is available either in annual hardback form or in a loose-leaf book that offers monthly updates. It contains information on all drugs and drug classes and is more up to date than a PDR. Another popular source is the *USP-DI (United States Pharmacopeia – Drug Information)*.

A pharmacist can always be asked about the specific drug, and the drug's package insert may provide needed information. Package inserts commonly list many of the same types of information found in the PDR and USP, including indications for use, mechanisms of action, contraindications, warnings, precautions, drug interactions, adverse reactions or effects, dosage information, and overdosage treatment information.

DRUG CLASSIFICATIONS

Drugs can be classified by group as follows:

- Drugs used to treat or prevent disease, such as hormones and vaccines.

- Drugs with a principal action on the body, such as analgesics and anti-inflammatory drugs.

- Drugs that act on specific systems or organs, such as respiratory and cardiovascular drugs.

- Drug preparations, such as suppositories, liquids, solids, topicals, etc.

Table 2-1 shows common drug classifications.

TABLE 2-1 Common Drug Classifications

Classification	Action	Examples
Analgesic	Relieves pain without causing loss of consciousness	acetaminophen, aspirin
Anesthetic	Produces numbness, either localized or generalized	lidocaine, procaine
Antacid	Neutralizes acid	Mylanta®, Milk of Magnesia®
Antianxiety	Relieves anxiety and muscle tension	diazepam, alprazolam
Antiarrhythmic	Controls cardiac arrhythmias	lidocaine, propranolol
Antibiotic	Destroys or inhibits growth of microorganisms	penicillins, cephalosporins
Anticholesterol	Reduces cholesterol	atorvastatin, simvastatin,
Anticoagulant	Prevents or delays blood clotting	coumarin, warfarin
Anticonvulsant	Prevents or relieves convulsions	carbamazepine, phenytoin
Antidepressant	Prevents or relieves symptoms of depression	amitriptyline, fluoxetine
Antidiarrheal	Prevents or relieves diarrhea	bismuth, diphenoxylate
Antiemetic	Prevents or relieves nausea and vomiting	dimenhydrinate, trimethobenzamide
Antihistamine	Counteracts histamine to combat allergy symptoms	diphenhydramine fexofenadine
Antihypertensive	Prevents or controls high blood pressure	methyldopa, metoprolol
Anti-inflammatory	Counteracts inflammation	ibuprofen, naproxen
Antineoplastic	Kills or destroys malignant cells	busulfan, cyclophosphamide
Antipsychotic	Helps in schizophrenia and chronic brain syndrome	chlorpromazine, haloperidol
Antipyretic	Reduces fever	acetaminophen, ibuprofen, aspirin (should not be used for fever in children)
Antitussive	Prevents or relieves coughing	codeine, dextromethorphan
Anti-ulcer	Relieves and heals ulcers by blocking hydrochloric acid	cimetidine, omeprazole
Bronchodilator	Dilates bronchi	albuterol, isoproterenol
Contraceptive	Prevents conception	ethinyl estradiol, norethindrone
Decongestant	Reduces nasal congestion or swelling	oxymetazoline, pseudoephedrine
Diuretic	Increases urine excretion	chlorothiazide, furosemide
Expectorant	Facilitates removal of secretions from mucous membranes	guaifenesin, iodinated glycerol
Hypnotic	Produces sleep or hypnosis	chloral hydrate, secobarbital
Hypoglycemic	Reduces blood glucose levels	insulin, tolbutamide
Laxative	Loosens and promotes normal bowel elimination	docusate sodium, psyllium
Muscle relaxant	Produces relaxation of skeletal muscle	methocarbamol, orphenadrine
Sedative	Produces a calming effect without causing sleep	amobarbital, phenobarbital
Tranquilizer	Reduces mental tension and anxiety	alprazolam, chlordiazepoxide
Vasodilator	Relaxes blood vessels and reduces blood pressure	atenolol, nitroglycerin
Vasopressor	Produces vessel contraction; increases blood pressure	metaraminol, norepinephrine

PRINCIPAL DRUG ACTIONS

Drugs differ widely in their actions, as listed below:

- Local action – Acting on the cells and tissues in the area of the body to which it is administered.

- Systemic action – Acting throughout the body's cells and tissues by being carried via the bloodstream.

- Microbial action – Antimicrobial; acting on microorganisms in the body.

- Selective action – Having different types of action, such as stimulants (which increase cell activity) and depressants (which decrease cell activity).

- Synergistic action – Increasing or counteracting the action of another drug.

The four principal processes that affect drug action depend on the patient, the form of the drug, its chemical composition, and how it is administered. These processes are listed below:

1. *Absorption* – The process of a drug passing into body fluids and tissues by means of diffusion or osmosis

2. *Distribution* – The process of transportation from the blood to the intended site of action, biotransformation, storage, and elimination

3. *Biotransformation* – The process of chemical alteration (metabolism) in the body

4. *Elimination* – The process of excretion from the body via the gastrointestinal tract, urinary system (kidneys), respiratory tract, skin, mucous membranes, and mammary glands

Every drug has the potential for causing unintended effects rather than those for which it was administered. Undesirable drug actions include:

1. *Adverse reactions or effects* – Unfavorable or harmful unintended drug actions, such as allergic reactions; a severe reaction (**anaphylaxis**) can occur that can manifest quickly and result in breathing difficulties, shock, loss of consciousness, and even death; many drugs cause gastrointestinal problems (including pain, nausea, vomiting, and ulcers), headaches, and insomnia; less serious adverse effects are commonly called "side effects," and may include drowsiness and dizziness.

2. *Drug interactions* – The undesirable or desirable increasing (**potentiation**) or diminishing of another drug's actions; drugs may also interact with foods, tobacco, alcohol, and other substances.

It is vital that a patient's history of allergies be documented and verifie before dispensing or administering any medication. One or two injections c epinephrine usually reverse most occurrences of anaphylaxis, but transfer t an emergency room may be required for the proper care of the patient.

DRUG ROUTES

A drug's route refers to how it is to be administered. Some drugs hav multiple routes with which they can be administered, with the correct rout determined by the medication's action. Most injected medications reach th systemic circulation rapidly and quickly become effective, as do sublingua medications (such as nitroglycerin). Oral medications act more slowl because they must first be dissolved in the stomach and then absorbed int the bloodstream. Suppositories are absorbed more slowly than injected an sublingual medications.

A patient's physical condition, emotional state, and level c consciousness are all considered when selecting the proper rout of administration. Drug characteristics are also important to know an understand. For example, insulin is usually given by injection because is (in most formulations) destroyed by digestive enzymes, prohibiting ora administration. Insulin is also available as a nasal spray.

The most frequently used routes of administration are oral an parenteral routes. It should be noted that while the term **parenteral** actuall means "by means other than the digestive tract," it is commonly thought of a being defined by the term "injectable." Parenteral administration is associate with all forms of a drug administered by a syringe, needle, or cathete (including intramuscular, subcutaneous, and intravenous administration Other common routes of administration include:

- Topical – direct application to the skin. Certain administrations c eye or ear medicines (liquid drops) may be referred to as "instillation though these are in fact topical routes.

- Sublingual – absorption under the tongue through the mucou membranes.

- Buccal – absorption into the mucous membranes between the cheek and gums.

- Rectal – absorption into the bloodstream via the rectum.

- Vaginal – absorption into the bloodstream via the vagina.

- Inhalation – the breathing in of sprays and aerosols through th mouth or nose.

Exercise

Objective: To become familiar with reading drug labels.

Read the following 10 drug labels and write down their various methods of administration (note: they may have more than one).

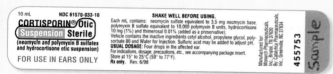

(Courtesy of Monarch Pharmaceuticals)

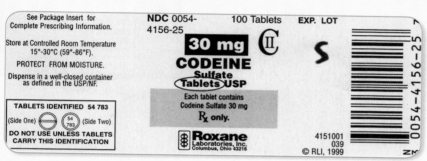

(Courtesy of Roxane Laboratories, Inc.)

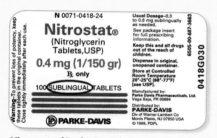

(Courtesy of Parke-Davis)

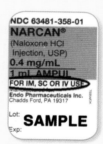

(Courtesy of Endo Pharmaceuticals)

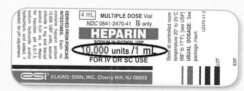

(Courtesy of Elkins-Sinn, Inc.)

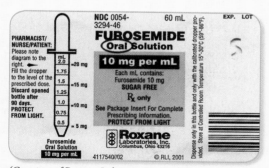

(Courtesy of Roxane Laboratories, Inc.)

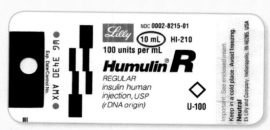

(Courtesy of Eli Lilly)

Exercise (Continued)

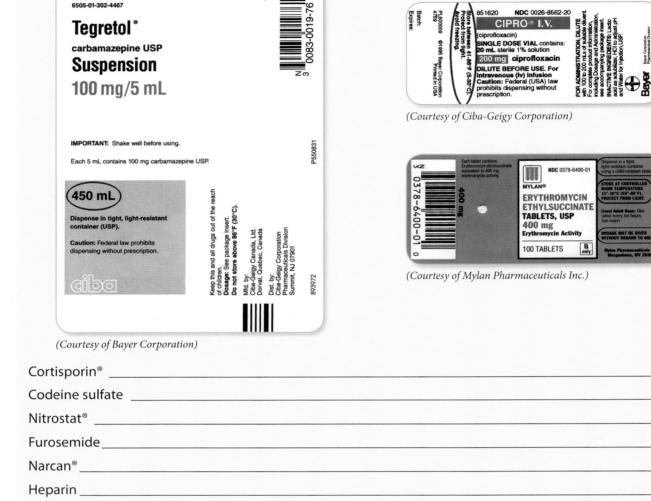

NDC 0083-0019-76   FSC 1841
6505-01-302-4467

Tegretol®

carbamazepine USP

Suspension

100 mg/5 mL

3 0083-0019-76 1

IMPORTANT: Shake well before using.

Each 5 mL contains 100 mg carbamazepine USP.

450 mL

Dispense in tight, light-resistant container (USP).

Caution: Federal law prohibits dispensing without prescription.

ciba

Keep this and all drugs out of the reach of children.
Dosage: See package insert.
Do not store above 86° F (30°C).

Mfd. by:
Ciba-Geigy Canada, Ltd.
Dorval, Quebec, Canada

Dist. by:
Ciba-Geigy Corporation
Pharmaceuticals Division
Summit, NJ 07901

P550831

893972

(Courtesy of Bayer Corporation)

851620   NDC 0026-8562-20

CIPRO® I.V.

(ciprofloxacin)

SINGLE DOSE VIAL contains:
20 mL sterile 1% solution
200 mg ciprofloxacin

DILUTE BEFORE USE. For
Intravenous (iv) Infusion
Caution: Federal (USA) law
prohibits dispensing without
prescription.

Store between 41-86°F (5-30°C).
Protect from light.
Avoid freezing.

PLS00009
4759

©1995 Bayer Corporation
Printed in USA

Batch:
Expires:

FOR ADMINISTRATION, DILUTE
with 100 to 200 mLs of suitable diluent.
For complete product information,
including Dosage and Administration,
see accompanying package insert.
INACTIVE INGREDIENTS: Lactic
acid as solution, HCl to adjust pH
and Water for Injection, USP.

Bayer Corporation
Pharmaceutical Division
400 Morgan Lane
West Haven, CT 06516

Bayer

(Courtesy of Ciba-Geigy Corporation)

Each tablet contains:
Erythromycin ethylsuccinate
equivalent to 400 mg
erythromycin activity.

NDC 0378-6400-01

MYLAN®

**ERYTHROMYCIN
ETHYLSUCCINATE
TABLETS, USP**

400 mg
Erythromycin Activity

100 TABLETS   R only

0378-6400-01

400 mg

Dispense in a tight,
light-resistant container
using a child-resistant closure.

**STORE AT CONTROLLED
ROOM TEMPERATURE
15°-30°C (59°-86°F).
PROTECT FROM LIGHT.**

Usual Adult Dose: One
tablet every six hours.
See insert.

**DOSAGE MAY BE GIVEN
WITHOUT REGARD TO MEALS.**

Mylan Pharmaceuticals Inc.
Morgantown, WV 26505

RM6400A5

(Courtesy of Mylan Pharmaceuticals Inc.)

Cortisporin® _____

Codeine sulfate _____

Nitrostat® _____

Furosemide _____

Narcan® _____

Heparin _____

Humulin R® _____

Cipro® _____

Tegretol® _____

Erythromycin _____

DRUG FORMS

Solids, semisolids, and liquids are the three basic types of dru
preparations. Some drugs are soluble in water, while others are soluble i
alcohol or in a mixture of solvents. Oral drugs are commonly in the form
of tablets, capsules, caplets, liquids, and powders (which are usually mixe

with a liquid solvent). Injectable drugs must be in the form of a liquid, but may need to be mixed with a liquid solvent beginning with a powder base. Common drug forms are explained below:

- Solid and semisolid preparations – offer easy dispensing of many different dosages; include tablets, capsules, caplets, troches or lozenges, suppositories, and ointments.

- Liquid preparations – contain drugs that have been dissolved or suspended; include suspensions, aerosols, mists, emulsions, elixirs, fluidextracts, and spirits.

- Transdermal preparations – adhesive patches transfer a drug through the skin; these commonly include medications for motion sickness, angina pectoris, menopausal symptoms, smoking cessation, and contraception.

- Inhalation medications – often administered by inhalation devices, these are used for bronchodilation, hypoxia, cardiovascular collapse, congestive heart failure, and pneumonia.

- Implantation – implantable devices placed beneath the skin near blood vessels that lie below; may be used to treat conditions such as cancer and diabetes, or for contraception; greater doses with fewer adverse effects than by systemic routes can be delivered.

Alert!

Expiration dates should be checked carefully before a drug is compounded, dispensed, or administered.

Exercise

Objective: To become familiar with reading drug labels.

Refer back to each of the labels presented in the previous exercise. List the drug forms for each.

Cortisporin _____

Codeine sulfate_____

Nitrostat _____

Furosemide_____

Narcan_____

Heparin _____

Humulin R _____

Cipro _____

Tegretol_____

Erythromycin _____

STORAGE AND HANDLING

The storage and handling of medications should always involv precautions that focus on the types of medications in question. Medication should be stored in different ways. For example, some medications should b kept in their original containers on labeled shelves, while others may be kep in locked cabinets, darkened areas or containers (if they are light-sensitive) or in refrigerators if needed. They should be organized by their classification or alphabetically. Certain medications need to be kept in glass container because they may react with containers made of plastic. Storage requirement are usually listed on each drug label. Medications intended for internal us must be kept separate from those intended for external use. Expiration date must always be checked, with outdated medications disposed of properly.

Alert!

Generally, medications should not be exposed to sunlight, bright lights, moisture, or extremes in temperature.

Exercise

Objective: To become familiar with reading drug labels.

Once again, refer to the labels presented on pages 43-44. Write down the proper storage of each of the drugs as indicated on their labels.

Cortisporin _____

Codeine sulfate _____

Nitrostat _____

Furosemide _____

Heparin _____

Humulin R _____

Tegretol _____

Erythromycin _____

Alert!

After compounding, attention is given to issues surrounding the correct storage of drugs so that they maintain their effectiveness, including the specific needs of more sensitive drugs.

PROPER DRUG DISPOSAL

Alert!

Tetracycline has been shown to cause kidney damage, in some cases leading to death, when used after its expiration date.

Drugs that have reached their printed **expiration dates** must be remove from stock shelves and destroyed. They cannot be dispensed due to potentia harmful effects. Though most drugs become less potent after their expiratio dates, some, such as cough syrups, can actually become more potent becaus of evaporation of their alcohol content.

There are different ways of disposing of expired drugs, depending o their form. Certain liquids, ointments, and powdered drugs can be rinse down a drain until they disappear completely from view. Vials and ampoule of some liquid drugs may also be poured down drains. Certain pills an capsules can be flushed down toilet systems—this information is include in their packaging. Medications that have been removed from their original containers should never be re-used by anyone.

When a pharmacist discovers that a large amount of drugs in inventory is soon to expire, these drugs should be returned to the manufacturer or wholesaler 1 month prior to the expiration date. In this way, the pharmacy can receive credit for these drugs and not be fully charged for them as it would be once the expiration date is reached. An example is immunoglobulin, which is commonly returned 1 month before expiration. Wholesalers commonly offer to properly dispose of expired drugs.

Any controlled substance (Schedule II drug) that has expired must be disposed of in the manner described on its packaging. Any of these substances that have been dropped or spilled require the completion of proper documentation of the accident. Losses or thefts of controlled substances must be reported to the local DEA office as well as the local police, along with appropriate paperwork being completed explaining the occurrence.

Exercise

Objective: To become familiar with reading drug labels.

The following tetracycline label indicates that the medication has reached its expiration date.

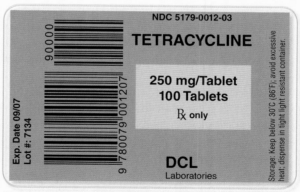

(Courtesy of Bristol-Myers Squibb)

List the sources where you may find disposal information for this product.

_____

_____

Research and describe the proper method of disposing of this medication.

_____

_____

_____

_____

EMERGENCY DRUGS AND SUPPLIES

Emergency drugs should be kept in specific trays, boxes, cabinets, or crash carts. A list of drugs that should be kept on hand for emergencies is shown in Table 2-2.

TABLE 2-2   Commonly Used Emergency Drugs

Generic Name	Trade Name	Uses
albuterol	Proventil®	A bronchodilator; relaxes smooth muscle of the respiratory tract
chlorothiazide	Diuril®	Promotes urine excretion
dextrose	(generic only)	Used for hypoglycemia to counteract hyperinsulinism
diazepam	Valium®	A muscle relaxant; used for antianxiety, to calm anxious patients and relax muscles; is a Schedule IV drug and must be kept in a locked cabinet
digoxin	Lanoxin®	A cardiac drug; used for CHF, arrhythmias; it slows and strengthens heartbeat
diphenhydramine	Benadryl®	An antihistamine; relieves allergic symptoms
epinephrine	Adrenalin®	A vasoconstrictor; relieves anaphylactic shock
hydrocortisone	Cortef®	An anti-inflammatory; used to suppress swelling and shock
insulin	Terumo, BD®	To prevent diabetic coma
naloxone	Narcan®	An antidote; used for narcotic overdose
nitroglycerin	Nitrogard®	A vasodilator; it dilates coronary arteries and is used in the treatment of angina pectoris
prochlorperazine	Compazine®	An antiemetic; relieves symptoms of nausea and vomiting
verapamil	Calan®	Used for cardiac arrhythmia; stable and unstable angina

Supplies and equipment that should be kept on an emergency cart include:

- Airways
- Alcohol
- Constriction bands
- Defibrillators
- IV fluid medications

- IV tape
- IV tubing
- Needles
- Oxygen and oxygen masks
- Personal protective equipment
- Sphygmomanometer
- Stethoscope
- Suction equipment (nasopharyngeal)
- Swabs
- Syringes

All equipment should be checked on a regular basis for functionality and freshness. This may be weekly or monthly depending on use. Used items should be replaced promptly and expired drugs and supplies must be discarded upon reaching their expiration date. The checking of updating of supplies must be documented in writing.

Exercise

Objective: To become familiar with the components on a variety of crash carts.

Compare and contrast adult, pediatric, and neonatal emergency carts.

SUMMARY

State law governs the practice of prescribing medications for patients. Both legend and OTC drugs have the potential to cause harm if not taken exactly as directed. Drugs must be used before their expiration dates, stored properly, and disposed of correctly after they expire. Information about the qualities and strengths of drugs can be found in drug standards and references known as the United States Pharmacopoeia/National Formulary, Physician's Desk Reference (PDR), drug package inserts, and others. Every drug can cause unintended effects, and knowledge of drug classifications, actions, routes, and forms is essential for the practicing pharmacy technician.

REVIEW QUESTIONS

Multiple Choice

1. The pink section of the PDR lists which of the following?

    A. classifications of drugs
    B. alphabetical drug manufacturers
    C. brand and generic names
    D. over-the-counter drugs

2. Unfavorable drug actions are called:

    A. drug interactions
    B. adverse reactions
    C. medication errors
    D. synergistic actions

3. Which of the following drugs may be administered to treat an anaphylactic condition?

    A. penicillin
    B. disulfiram
    C. epinephrine
    D. scopolamine

4. Medications designed to absorb into the mucous membranes between the cheeks and gums are called:

    A. buccal
    B. topical
    C. sublingual
    D. all of the above

5. When a drug is administered by a syringe, needle, or catheter, it is called:

    A. instillation
    B. implantation
    C. parenteral
    D. urethral

6. According to drug classifications, which of the following drugs is an anticoagulant?

    A. lidocaine
    B. ibuprofen
    C. atenolol
    D. coumarin

7. Which of the following types of drugs is designed to reduce fever?

    A. decongestant
    B. antitussive
    C. antipyretic
    D. antiemetic

8. Prescription drugs are also called:

   A. controlled substances
   B. legend drugs
   C. over-the-counter drugs
   D. none of the above

9. Which of the following is an example of a diuretic?

   A. busulfan
   B. methyldopa
   C. methocarbamol
   D. furosemide

10. A drug whose action causes an increase in the action of another drug is said to have this type of effect.

   A. synergistic
   B. systemic
   C. microbial
   D. local

Matching

Classification of Drugs

1. _____ Antibiotic

2. _____ Antacid

3. _____ Anesthetic

4. _____ Antihypertensive

5. _____ Anti-inflammatory

6. _____ Hypnotic

Examples
   A. ibuprofen
   B. procaine
   C. methyldopa
   D. secobarbital
   E. Mylanta
   F. tetracycline

Fill in the Blank

1. Ointments and powders can be disposed of by _____ down a drain until they disappear completely from view.

2. The PDR is one of the most widely used _____ books.

3. All controlled substances are listed in the PDR with the symbol _____ followed by a Roman numeral.

4. The process of chemical alteration in the body is referred to as _____.

5. Absorption into the mucous membranes between the cheeks and gums is called _____ administration.

6. The process of transportation from the blood to the intended site of action, biotransformation, storage, and elimination is known as _____.

Identification of Prescription Components

Examine the following prescription. Label these components of the prescription.

A. The superscription
B. The inscription
C. The subscription
D. The signa
E. Prescriber information
F. Patient information

COMMUNITY MEDICAL CLINIC
1700 South Tamiami Trail, Sarasota, FL 34239.   (813) 952-2577

Patient Name: *Mary Chase* _____ Date: _12-10-xx_

Address: _____

℞   *Cephalexin 250 mg* _____

28 _____

Tgid _____

Private Pay
Private Insurance
Medicaid
CMC

Refill: _0_   Physician Signature: *J. Brown* _____ M.D.

Physician Name (printed): ___J. Brown___

Physician DEA#: _____

Delmar/Cengage Learning

Introduction to Compounding

OBJECTIVES

Upon completion of this chapter, the student should be able to:

1. Explain why compounding is becoming more common in pharmacy practice.
2. Describe the various types of compounding.
3. Discuss the roles of pharmacists with ambulatory care patients.
4. List five compounding factors that affect the quality of drug products.
5. Explain the role of pharmacy technicians in compounding.

GLOSSARY

Ambulatory care compounding – This type of compounding is designed for non-institutionalized patients; they may be outpatients or home-care patients.

Batch – A group of similarly prepared substances.

Batch-prepared prescriptions – Those in which multiple identical units are prepared in a single operation, in anticipation of the receipt of prescriptions.

Compounding – The preparation, mixing, assembling, packaging, or labeling of a drug or device as the result of a practitioner's prescription drug order.

Environment – A compounding environment consists of a separate area that is clean, neat, well-lit, and quiet; aseptic conditions are usually required.

Equipment – Compounding equipment includes clean air environments, electronic balances, ointment slabs, spatulas, mortars, pestles, electronic or manual capsule-making devices, glassware, and sterilization devices.

Formulas – Standards for compounding that ensure batch-to-batch consistency, documentable procedures, and proper preparation methods and ingredients.

Hospital pharmacy compounding – Compounding of drug products within a pharmacy that is located inside a hospital; it can provide better care and cost savings both to the hospital and to patients.

Nuclear pharmacy compounding – This type of compounding focuses on radioactive drugs (radiopharmaceuticals) that are used for diagnosis and therapy.

Routine prescriptions – Those that pharmacists may expect to receive in the future on a routine basis; also called "maintenance prescriptions."

Shelf life – The length of time a drug remains potent.

Stability – Duration of chemical, physical, or microbiological properties of a substance that may be affected by temperature, light exposure, and specific container types.

OVERVIEW

Compounding is a basic component of the practice of pharmacy tha[t] combined with clinical functions offers balanced patient care. It is u[p] to the experience and expertise of each pharmacist to correctly adjus[t] dosage forms, frequencies, and quantities for each patient. The pharmac[y] technician must be aware of the various factors that affect the compoundin[g] of pharmaceuticals. The technician plays an assistive role in the preparatio[n] and dispensing of compounded medications.

Pharmaceutical compounding activities are increasing due to:

- a limited number of dosage forms,
- a limited number of drug strengths,
- shortages of drug products and combinations,
- orphan drugs,
- special patient populations,
- new therapeutic approaches, and
- the existence of environments such as home health care and hospice[.]

Compounding for specific, individual patients is becoming mor[e] common in pharmacy practice. Pharmacists who compound medication[s] develop unique patient relationships and must work closely with physician[s] to solve individual patient medication problems.

Batch (a group of similarly prepared substances) production of steril[e] products is also increasing, especially in the home health care and hospita[l] environments. This may be due in part to drug therapy pattern changes[,] self-administration of parenteral products, and the use of injectable dru[g] products in hospitals that are not currently commercially available.

WHAT IS COMPOUNDING?

According to the National Association of Boards of Pharmacy (NABP)[,] **compounding** (in simplified terms) means the "preparation, mixing[,] assembling, packaging, or labeling of a drug or device as the result of [a] practitioner's prescription drug order." It also includes the preparatio[n] of drugs and devices in anticipation of prescription drug orders base[d] on routine, regularly observed patterns. Compounding may involve ora[l] liquids, topical creams or ointments, suppositories, troches, conversion of dosage forms, preparation of dosage forms from bulk chemicals, preparation of intravenous (IV) admixtures, parenteral nutrition solutions, pediatric dosage forms, radioactive isotopes, and the preparation for use of various drug devices.

Routine prescriptions are those that pharmacists may expect to receive in the future on a consistent basis. Routine prescriptions may require that *standardized preparations* be made (requiring preparation protocols to be kept on file). Routine prescriptions are also known as "maintenance prescriptions." **Batch-prepared prescriptions** are those in which multiple identical units are prepared in a single operation, *in anticipation* of the receipt of prescriptions.

TYPES OF COMPOUNDING

The various types of compounding include hospital pharmacy compounding, ambulatory care compounding, and nuclear pharmacy compounding. Each of these areas has its own unique focus and specialization.

Hospital Pharmacy Compounding

Hospital pharmacy compounding can provide better care and cost savings both to the hospital and to patients. Improving outcomes and helping patients to go home as soon as they can should be the end goal of the hospital pharmacist as he or she works in conjunction with the hospital health care team. The products typically compounded by the hospital pharmacy include:

- daily intravenous medications
- total parenteral nutrition (TPN) solutions
- antibiotic piggybacks
- IV additives
- pediatric dosage forms

Hospital pharmacy policies and procedures must be documented in writing to establish guidelines for the proper conduct of compounding activities.

Ambulatory Care Compounding

Ambulatory care compounding is designed for patients who do not require a hospital stay. Most of these non-institutionalized patients are considered *outpatients*, though they may also be home-care patients. Most ambulatory patients are responsible for obtaining and administering their own medications. The roles of pharmacists with ambulatory care patient can include all of the following:

- Compliance enhancement
- Compounding
- Counseling
- Dispensing
- Minimizing expenditures
- Minimizing medication errors
- Therapeutic drug monitoring

Because compounded medications all have unique characteristic ambulatory patients must be counseled by their pharmacists. Ambulator patients must present their prescriptions themselves, or through thei caregiver. Pharmacy technicians may assist pharmacists in ambulator care compounding, dispensing, minimizing expenditures, and minimizin medication errors.

Nuclear Pharmacy Compounding

Nuclear pharmacy compounding focuses on radioactive drugs that ar used for diagnosis and therapy. Also known as *radiopharmaceuticals,* thes drugs are heavily regulated by the FDA because they contain an unstabl radioactive nucleus. They are designed for localized treatments in specifi tissues. The Nuclear Regulatory Commission is also involved in the regulatio of these drugs. Nuclear pharmacists and pharmacy technicians must receiv specialized training to work with these substances, which are usuall administered intravenously under aseptic conditions. This type of pharmac has grown in number very quickly in the last 25 years, and there are nov hundreds of professional nuclear pharmacists and specialized facilities.

The most common setting for the provision of radiopharmaceutical by nuclear pharmacists is a commercially centralized nuclear pharmacy Radiopharmaceuticals are generally prepared early in the morning, and unit dose are then delivered to hospitals in the region surrounding the nuclear pharmacy.

COMPOUNDING FACTORS

The factors that are important to consider when compounding includ stability, equipment, environment, formulas, and chemical supplies.

Stability

Stability may be chemical, physical, or microbiological. A chemica substance is considered "stable" if it is not reactive during normal use, an keeps its potency over the pre-determined period of time it will be used

The length of time that a drug remains potent is referred to as its **shelf life**. Compounded products are assigned a *beyond-use date* instead of an *expiration date*. Beyond-use dates must be determined using documented literature about the drug's stability (via laboratory testing or the manufacturer). The pharmacist should use professional judgment as well. Stability may be affected by storage conditions that include temperature, exposure to light, and specific container types. Many compounded drugs, which are generally reconstituted, have a beyond-use date ranging between 30 days and 1 year. They should be refrigerated (between 2 and 8°C), but not frozen. Water-containing formulations made from ingredients in solid form (when properly stored, usually at cold temperatures) should not be used after 14 days.

Equipment

Equipment used in compounding includes clean air environments, electronic balances, ointment slabs, spatulas, mortars, pestles, electronic or manual capsule-making devices, glassware, and sterilization devices. Today's compounding equipment has changed greatly. The additions of ultrafreezers to replace standard refrigerator/freezers are one common upgrade that has helped increase the effectiveness of compounded products.

Environment

The **environment** for compounding consists of a separate area that is clean, neat, and well lit. For sterile products, a clean air environment consisting of laminar airflow hoods and isolation barriers must be used, except in an emergency. In emergencies, only pharmacists, nurses, or doctors may compound outside of the clean air environment.

Formulas

As a result of the requirement of consistency when compounding, **formulas** (standards of compounding) should be strictly adhered to in assuring that the proper preparation methods and ingredients are used for each compounded product. These standards ensure batch-to-batch consistency and a documented process of workflow to reduce future errors. Documentation can be made on formula worksheets or "logs." Reviews of the techniques used in compounding may be made regularly to improve quality.

A *master formula sheet* may be used to document information about each formulation that is used in the pharmacy. These sheets commonly contain information about the ingredients of a formulation, its manufacturer, lot number, the manufacturer's expiration date, the formula quantity, the quantity used, the date it was prepared, the person who formulated the mixture, and the person who checked it for accuracy. These sheets usually contain the required equipment for formulating, manufacturing directions, description of the final appearance of the mixture, information that wil appear on its label, and a description of the length it will be stable.

Chemicals and Supplies

Proper vehicles (such as creams or ointments) as well as active ingredient (usually powders or chemicals) are required for effective compounding Proper dispensing containers that will not compromise the effectivenes of the products must be used to hold the compounded products that ar created. Compounding pharmacists use chemicals that come from reliabl commercial sources that are regulated by various governmental agencie Suppliers of compounding chemicals and substances should suppl certificates of analysis that prove the purity and quality of their product Only manufactured drugs that bear lot numbers and expiration dates ma be accepted as potential sources of active ingredients.

It is the job of the pharmacist to select the most appropriate qualitie of chemicals for compounding. They should begin by using the United State Pharmacopoeia/National Formulary to make their initial choices, and kee certificates of analysis on file for each chemical that they use in their pharmacy

ROLE OF PHARMACY TECHNICIANS IN COMPOUNDING

The pharmacy technician's role in compounding is always changin and expanding. Most commonly, pharmacy technicians are involved in th compounding of intravenous (IV) piggybacks and large-volume parentera admixtures. It should be noted that IV piggybacks (IVPBs) are often als called "minibags." They may also be involved with unit dose injections an total parenteral nutrition solutions. On a lesser scale, they work with narcoti infusions and chemotherapy agents.

Pharmacy technicians may participate in all of the following:

- The securing of all prescribed medications or devices from inventory
- Measuring finished dosage forms (known as "quality sufficient" or "q.s.")
- Collecting ingredients for sterile preparations.
- Determining amounts of ingredients to be compounded.
- Compounding sterile preparations using appropriate asepti technique, equipment, and devices.
- Compounding cytotoxic or other hazardous preparations.
- Disposing of hazardous or non-hazardous waste materials.
- Packaging of finished preparations.
- Generating accurate and complete labels and affixing then appropriately.
- Storing all medications correctly prior to dispensing.

Summary

Compounding for specific, individual patients is becoming more common in pharmacy practice. Pharmacists or technicians must be trained in advance for compounding procedures and follow state and federal laws and guidelines.

Compounding means the "preparation, mixing, assembling, packaging, or labeling of a drug or device as the result of a practitioner's prescription drug order." The various types of compounding include hospital pharmacy compounding, ambulatory care compounding, and nuclear compounding.

There are various factors that may affect compounding. These factors include stability of substances, equipment, environment, formulas, chemicals, and supplies.

Most commonly, pharmacy technicians are involved in the compounding of intravenous (IV) piggybacks and large-volume parenteral admixtures. They may also be involved with unit dose injections and total parenteral nutrition solutions. On a lesser scale, technicians work with narcotic infusions and chemotherapy agents.

Review Questions

Multiple Choice

1. The performance of assembling, mixing, preparing, and labeling is called:

    A. standardizing
    B. dispensing
    C. bulk chemical mixing
    D. compounding

2. Nuclear pharmacy compounding focuses on which of the following products?

    A. depressant drugs
    B. radioactive drugs
    C. microbiological agents
    D. chemical powders

3. Water-containing formulations that are properly stored should be used before:

    A. 4 days
    B. 14 days
    C. 4 weeks
    D. 14 weeks

4. Which of the following statements is correct regarding the roles of pharmacy technicians in compounding?

    A. They are never involved in compounding.
    B. The state board of pharmacy only allows trained pharmacists to do compounding.
    C. Their roles are always changing and expanding.
    D. None of the above are correct.

5. Which of the following is *not* a role of a pharmacist as related to ambulatory care patients?

    A. compounding
    B. administering medications
    C. therapeutic drug monitoring
    D. minimizing expenditures

6. Compounded products are assigned:

    A. an expiration date
    B. a beyond-use date
    C. an exposure to light ratio
    D. an exposure to heat ratio

7. For aseptic conditions, a clean air environment consists of:

    A. laminar airflow hoods
    B. isolation patients
    C. isolation barriers
    D. A and C

8. Pharmacy technicians may participate in which of the following?

    A. collecting ingredients for sterile preparation
    B. determining amounts of ingredients to be compounded
    C. compounding cytotoxic preparations
    D. all of the above

9. Which of the following compounding medications may be involved in hospital pharmacy?

    A. total parenteral nutrition
    B. IV additives
    C. antibiotic piggybacks
    D. all of the above

10. Ambulatory care compounding is designed for which of the following patients?

    A. long-term care patients
    B. hospice patients
    C. inpatients
    D. non-institutionalized patients

Matching

1. _____ Designed for patients who are not institutionalized

2. _____ Adhered to in order to assure that the proper preparation methods and ingredients for each compounded product are used

3. _____ Multiple identical units are prepared in a single operation

4. _____ Work closely with physicians to solve individual patient medication problems

5. _____ Focuses on the compounding of radiopharmaceuticals

6. _____ Typically provides daily intravenous medications

    A. Hospital pharmacy compounding
    B. Pharmacists
    C. Nuclear pharmacy compounding
    D. Batch-prepared prescriptions
    E. Formulas
    F. Ambulatory care compounding

Fill in the Blank

1. Radioactive drugs are also known as _____.

2. For aseptic conditions, a clean air environment consists of laminar _____.

3. Intermittent intravenous preparations of secondary solutions are called _____.

4. Preparation, mixing, and assembling of drugs or devices is called _____.

Short Answer

1. Write a simple definition of the term "compounding."

2. Make a list of the common products compounded in the hospital pharmacy.

3. List the most common types of compounding.

4. List all the factors about compounding that you have learned and define each of them.

5. List the various roles of pharmacy technicians in compounding.

REFERENCES

http://www.nmcpr.state.nm.us (Click on "NMAC"; "Browse Compilation"; "Occupational and Professional Licensing"; "Pharmacists"; "Compounding of Non-Sterile Pharmaceuticals")

NONSTERILE COMPOUNDING PRODUCTS

CHAPTER 4

Equipment and Supplies for Nonsterile Compounding

OBJECTIVES

Upon completion of this chapter, the student should be able to:

1. Name the 10 most common and important types of equipment for extemporaneous compounding and their indications.

2. Identify the different types of graduates and demonstrate how to correctly read the amount in a graduate.

3. Describe beakers, beaker tongs, and their indications.

4. Perform correct weighing of 1 g and 5 g of a powder using a Class A prescription balance.

5. Explain the advantages of ultrasonic cleaners and when they should be used.

6. Describe the indications of hot plates in the pharmacy.

7. Explain and demonstrate the use of heat sealers.

8. Demonstrate the donning and wearing of safety equipment for compounding in order to prevent the transfer of pathogens to and from the staff.

GLOSSARY

Class A prescription balance – The most commonly used balance by pharmacists; it is a one- or two-pan torsion balance that may be digital (electronic weight sensing) or spring-based in design; the two-pan type requires the use of external weights for measurements exceeding 1 g.

Cavitation – The rapid swelling and collapsing of microscopic bubbles.

Compounding slab – A hard, non-absorbable flat surface used for the compounding of different medications or substances; usually made of ground glass.

Conical graduate – A container that resembles a cone—hence the name—with a wider top that tapers down to a thinner base; it has graduated markings for measuring liquids.

Dry Baths

Brushes

Tongs

Crimpers

Decappers

Suppository Molds

Ultrasonic Cleaners

Pipettes and Pipette Fillers

Spray Bottles

Glass Stirring Rods

Graduates

Droppers

Beakers

Beaker Tongs

Funnels

Capsule-Filling Equipment

Tablet Molds

Carts

Refrigerators and Freezers

Safety Glasses, Gloves, and Masks

Counter balance – A double-pan balance designed to weigh large quantities of bulk products.

Cylindrical graduate – A container that is cylindrical in shape, with the top being of the same circumference as the base; it also has graduated markings for measuring liquids.

Electronic balance – A scale that uses electronic components and digital readouts to calibrate the weighing of different substances; electronic balances are most frequently used now.

Forceps – Used to pick up prescription weights and ensure that oil is not deposited on the weight.

Glassine paper – Used underneath substances to be weighed to keep them from soiling balance pans; today, weighing boats are preferred over glassine paper.

Meniscus – The bottom portion of the concave surface of a liquid that is used to measure the volume of the liquid in a container such as a *graduate.*

Mortar – A vessel with a rounded interior in which drugs or other substances are crushed by means of a pestle.

Pestle – An instrument in the shape of a rod with one end that is rounded and weighted; used for crushing and mixing substances in a mortar.

Pipette – Also spelled "pipet," this is a graduated tube (marked in mL) used to transport a certain volume of a liquid or gas.

Triturate – Reducing particle size within a mortar and pestle.

OVERVIEW

The correct equipment and supplies are important when compounding. Equipment used in the compounding of drug products must be of appropriate design, of adequate size, and suitably located to facilitate operations for the intended use, as well as for cleaning and maintenance. Therefore, pharmacy technicians should be familiar with those pieces of equipment that are necessary for compounding drugs. Many state boards of pharmacy have a required minimum list of equipment for compounding prescriptions. These pieces of equipment vary according to the amount of material needed and the type of compounded prescription. There are several conventional pieces of equipment and instruments that a pharmacist or pharmacy technician may use for the operation of compounding. This chapter presents a wide variety of different types of equipment that may be required for compounding because each pharmacy may have its own unique needs.

CLASS A PRESCRIPTION BALANCE

Each pharmacy is required to have a **Class A prescription balance** which may be an **electronic balance** (see Figure 4-1) or a spring-based balance (see Figure 4-2). Today, most pharmacies use electronic balances with digital readouts. Spring-based Class A balances have a weighing capacity that ranges from 6 mg to a maximum of 120 g. Digital (electronic) Class A balances have a weighing capacity that ranges from 1 mg to a maximum of 300 g. Class A balances are considered the most accurate class of balance used in the pharmacy. This piece of equipment may have one or two balances. They may be used for weighing small amounts of drugs. Electronic balances use electrical components and digital readouts to determine the weights of substances. Isopropyl alcohol is commonly used to clean balances after each procedure.

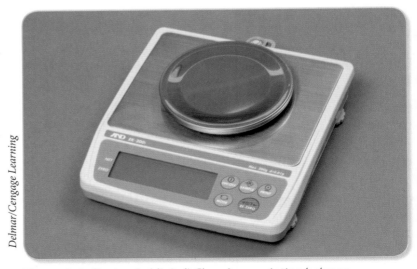

Delmar/Cengage Learning

Figure 4-1 Electronic (digital) Class A prescription balance.

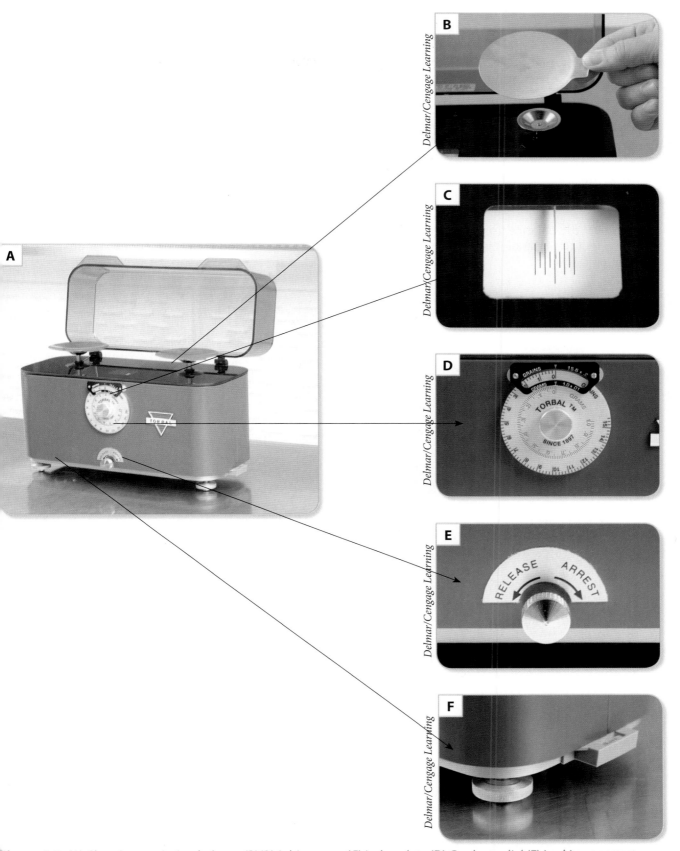

Figure 4-2 (A) Class A prescription balance (B) Weighing pans (C) Index plate (D) Graduate dial (E) Locking or arrest mechanism (F) Leveling feet.

Procedure: Calibrating a Class A Prescription Balance (both spring-based and electronic)

Objective: To properly set the calibration on a Class A prescription balance to ensure accurate measurement of materials.

Equipment Needed: Class A prescription balance

Step 1: First, "arrest" the balance by turning the *arrest knob* (Figure 4-3A).

Step 2: Level the balance from front to back by turning the *leveling screw feet* all the way in, and move them until all four sides of the balance are at the same distance from the surface they are resting upon (Figure 4-3B).

Step 3: Turn the *calibrated dial* to "zero," which sets the internal weights to zero (see Figure 4-3C).

Step 4: Level the balance from left to right by adjusting the *leveling screw feet*. This is done by rotating the screw feet until the unit is level (this is signified by the pointer resting at the center of the index). (See Figure 4-3D.)

Figure 4-3 Calibrating a spring-based balance. (A) Arrest the balance (B) Level the balance (C) Turn calibrated dial to zero (D) Level the balance.

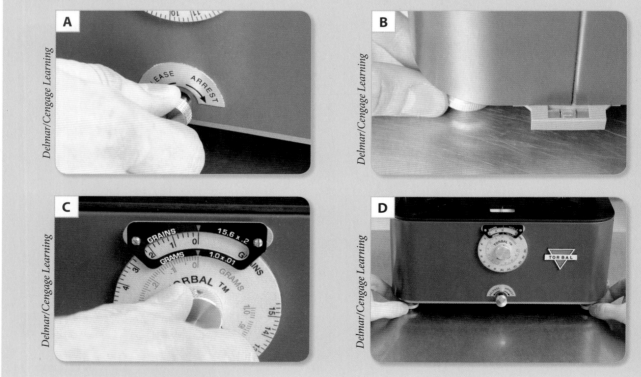

Electronic balance

Step 1: Turn the unit on, allowing it to "warm up" for a specified period.

Step 2: Press the "calibration" button while nothing is on the balance. The balance will then display a calibration mass amount that is needed.

Step 3: Place the predetermined amount of weight onto the weighing platform, and then depress the "calibration" button on the keypad. The unit is then calibrated and ready to use.

Procedure : Using a Class A Prescription Balance

Objective: To properly use a Class A prescription balance to measure materials.

Equipment Needed: Class A prescription balance, weighing boat or weighing paper, weights, material to weigh.

Step 1: Make sure the unit has been calibrated.

Step 2: Make sure that the balance is locked.

Step 3: Place a weighing boat or paper on each pan (Figure 4-4A).

Step 4: Unlock the balance by releasing the *arrest knob* (Figure 4-4B).

Step 5: Make sure that the pointer is resting at the center of the index (Figure 4-4C).

Step 6: Arrest the balance again.

Step 7: Place the required weights on the right pan (Figure 4-4D).

Step 8: Place the material you intend to weigh on the left pan (Figure 4-4E).

Step 9: Release the balance (Figure 4-4F).

Step 10: Notice to where the pointer moves. If it shifts to the left, there is too much material on the left pan (Figure 4-4G); if it shifts right, there is too little material on the left pan (Figure 4-4H).

Step 11: Remove or add material as needed by using a spatula, remembering to arrest the balance *each time* before material is removed or added (Figure 4-4I).

Step 12: Once the correct amount is on the left pan, double-check that you have weighed the correct amount and have used the correct weights (Figure 4-4J).

Figure 4-4 Use of a spring-based balance. (A) Place weighing paper on balance pan (B) Release the arrest knob.

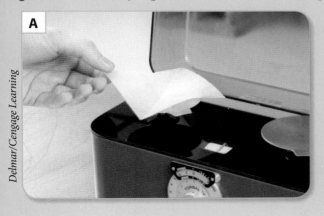

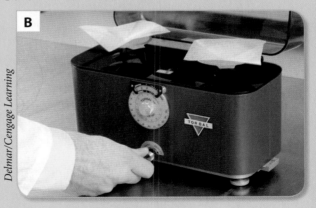

Delmar/Cengage Learning

Procedure: (Continued)

Figure 4-4 Use of a spring-based balance. (C) Verify the pointer is at center of the index (D) Place weights on right pan (E) Place material to be weighed on weighing paper on the left (F) Release the balance (G) If the pointer is too far left there is too much material on the pan (H) If the pointer is too far right there is too little material on the pan.

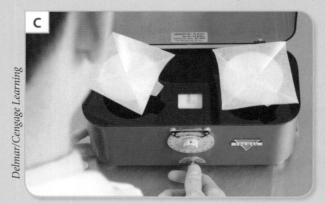

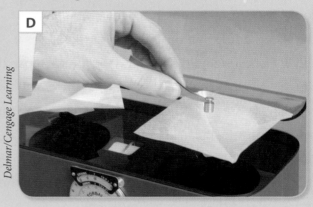

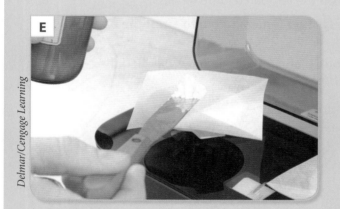

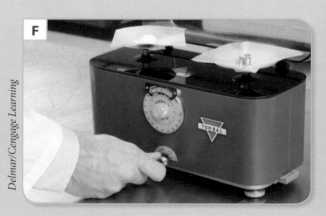

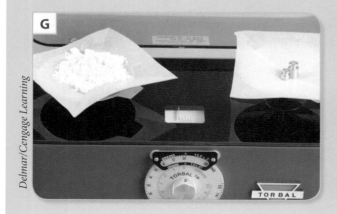

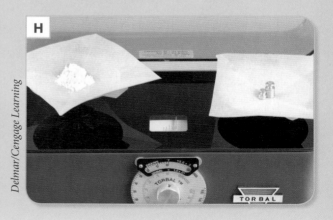

Procedure: (Continued)

Figure 4-4 Use of a spring-based balance. (I) Remove or add material until desired weight is reached (J) Double-check your measurements for accuracy.

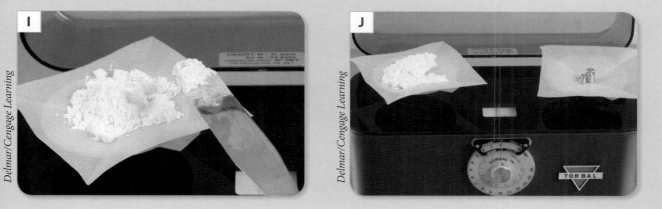

Exercise

Objective: To become proficient in the use of Class A prescription balances.

Demonstrate the procedures required for using balances and weights. Use a spring-based Class A prescription balance for this procedure. Weigh the following amounts: 1 mg, 10 mg, 55 mg, 150 mg, and 5 g.

Repeat the exercise using an electronic balance if available.

COUNTER BALANCES

A **counter balance** is capable of weighing larger quantities, up to about 5 kg. It is a double-pan balance. A counter balance is not indicated for prescription compounding. It is used for measuring bulk products. Counter balances should be calibrated by a professional calibration service. Isopropyl alcohol is commonly used to clean counter balances after each bulk product is weighed.

WEIGHTS

Good-quality weights are essential and they should be stored appropriately. Weights made from corrosion-resistant metals, such as brass, are preferred (Figure 4-5). Metric weights are kept in the front row of a standard weight rack and apothecary weights are kept in the back row. When transferring weights, always be careful not to drop them, and always use forceps. Weights can be cleaned with standard solutions designed for use with metals.

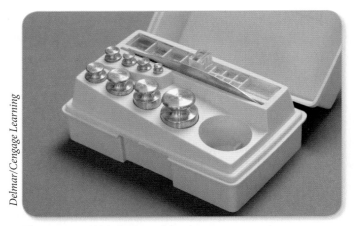

Figure 4-5 Weights used in pharmacy practice.

WEIGHING BOATS AND GLASSINE WEIGHING PAPER

Weighing boats (sometimes called "weighing dishes") are commonly diamond-shaped or square, and usually made of aluminum, plastic, o rubber (Figure 4-6). They are often used along with weighing papers tha help to keep surfaces clean from spills of powders or liquids (including dilute acids and alcohols). Weighing boats may be reusable or disposable and most commonly range from 1⅝ inches wide to 5½ inches wide, being up to 1 inch in depth. Most weighing boats are designed to withstand extreme temperatures. Reusable weighing boats may be cleaned with isopropyl alcohol or with cleaning solutions designed for aluminum.

Sheets of **glassine** "weighing" **paper** are used in the pharmacy fo keeping balance pans clean while weighing various substances (Figure 4-6) They have a smooth surface that is moisture-resistant and non-absorbent This paper is designed for single use and is therefore easily disposable Glassine paper is available in either square or rectangular shapes, and in a variety of sizes ranging between 3 and 6 inches per side. Weighing boats are used more frequently today than glassine paper.

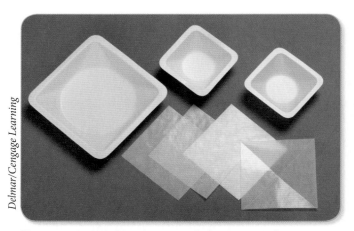

Figure 4-6 Weighing boats and glassine weighing paper.

Exercise

Objective: To become familiar with the equipment needed to properly weigh materials in pharmaceutical practice.

Practice using weighing boats and a Class A prescription balance to weigh the following amounts: 16 mg, 55 mg, and 60 g.

FORCEPS

Forceps are instruments with two blades and a handle, resembling scissors, that are used for handling, grasping, or compressing. Various types of forceps include alligator forceps (which feature angled "jaws"), tissue forceps (a type of tweezer), and hemostatic forceps (used for clamping blood vessels and other structures). Forceps may have straight, curved, or rounded tips (Figure 4-7). They have a variety of uses including dissection and the grasping and holding of a variety of specimens and pieces of equipment. They are usually made of stainless steel and may feature wood laminate sides. Forceps may be easily cleaned with alcohol and can be autoclaved.

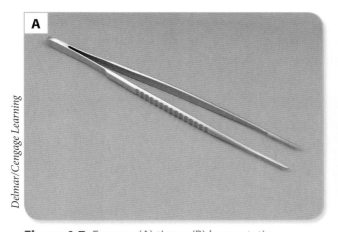
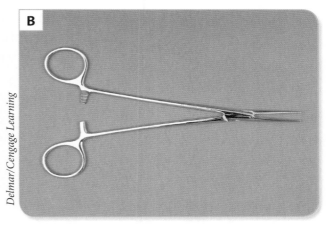

Delmar/Cengage Learning

Figure 4-7 Forceps (A) tissue (B) hemostatic.

SPATULAS

Spatulas are available in stainless steel, plastic, or hard rubber (Figure 4-8). Spatulas are used to transfer solid ingredients, such as ointments and creams, to weighing pans. Spatulas are also used to mix powders on an ointment slab. They must be clean and have indented edges. Spatulas may be cleaned with alcohol or detergents. Stainless steel spatulas may also be autoclaved.

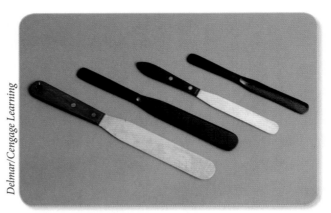

Figure 4-8 Spatulas.

Exercise

Objective: To become familiar with the use of a spatula.

Practice using a spatula to mix a powder with cocoa butter.

COMPOUNDING SLABS

The **compounding slab** is a plate made of ground glass or ceramic with a hard, flat, and non-absorbent surface for mixing compounds (Figure 4-9) Compounding slabs are also called ointment slabs because some ointment and creams are prepared on compounding slabs. Compounding slabs ma be easily cleaned with alcohol or detergents.

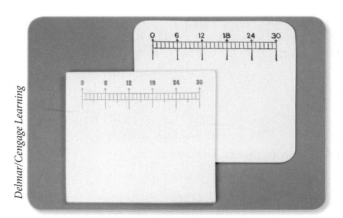

Figure 4-9 Compounding slab.

MORTARS AND PESTLES

A **mortar** is a cup-shaped vessel in which materials are ground or crushe by a **pestle** in the preparation of drugs. Pestles are rod-shaped instrument with one end that is rounded and weighted. Mortars and pestles are used t triturate (reduce particle size of) substances by grinding motions. Mortars and pestles are available in three types: glass (Figure 4-10A), Wedgwood, and porcelain (see Figure 4-10B), which is quite similar to Wedgwood in both use and appearance. Wedgwood and porcelain mortars and pestles are used to decrease particle size of solids to aid in dissolution in liquids and also to ensure comparable mixtures of semisolids and semisoft dosage forms. Certain emulsions must be compounded using Wedgwood and porcelain mortars and pestles because glass mortars and pestles will not allow the formation of stable emulsions. Glass mortars and pestles are preferred for mixing liquids and semisoft dosage forms. Advantages of glass mortars and pestles are that they are nonporous and nonstaining. Mortars and pestles may be easily cleaned with alcohol or detergents. However, it is important to make sure that the cleaning is thorough so that residue from drugs is fully removed prior to the next use.

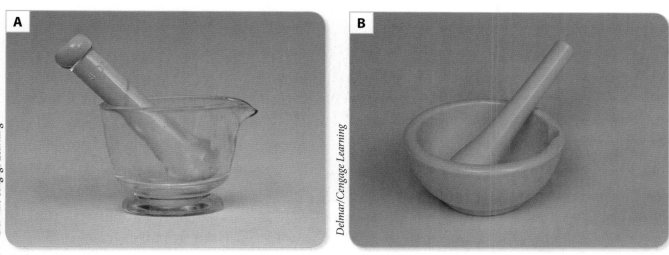

Delmar/Cengage Learning

Figure 4-10 (A) Glass mortar and pestle (B) Porcelain mortar and pestle.

Exercise

Objective: To become familiar with the proper uses of a mortar and pestle and the substances with which they can be used.

1. List two medications that should not be mixed with a Wedgwood or ceramic mortar and pestle. Explain why.

2. Put 10 sugar tablets into a mortar and use the pestle to grind them into a powder. Add them into a bottle of water for dilution.

ELECTRONIC MORTARS AND PESTLES

Electronic mortars and pestles (EMPs) have the ability to produce quality ointments, creams, and oral liquids. They use a spinning blade and moving arm to mix products, which can be weighed, mixed, and dispensed all in the same jar (see Figure 4-11). Electronic mortars and pestles are easily cleaned with alcohol or detergents, but should be maintained by an authorized service company.

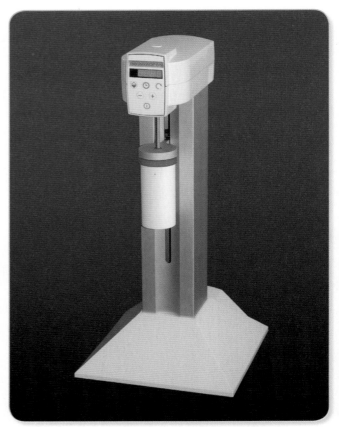

Figure 4-11 Electronic mortar and pestle. (Courtesy of Unguator USA, Norman, Oklahoma.)

BLENDERS

Blenders are used to thoroughly and accurately mix substances through rotational splitting. They also can be used to split or mix samples. There are generally two types of blenders, either high-energy or low-energy. Blenders may be easily cleaned by alcohol or detergents, but should be maintained by an authorized service company.

PROFESSIONAL MIXERS

Professional mixers provide fast, efficient, and thorough mixing and are available in a variety of different sizes. Some utilize acoustic fluidization also called "sonic mixing." Many of these mixers do not use blades, generate low heat, and keep contaminants out. Electronic mixers and blenders offer many advantages in compounding and are becoming increasingly popular.

for regular use. Professional mixers can be easily cleaned with alcohol or detergents, but should be maintained by an authorized service company.

HEAT GUNS

Heat guns are often used to shrink bands onto vials (see Figures 4-12A through 4-12D). This is accomplished by placing a shrinkable band onto a vial so that the medication label is clearly visible. The next step is to aim the heat gun (which resembles a hair dryer) at the vial, approximately 6 to 10 inches away. The vial should be turned several times to ensure that complete shrinking of the entire band is achieved. Heat guns can also shrink bands onto vials when several vials are placed into a tray at one time. Heat guns can easily be cleaned with isopropyl alcohol. They should be regularly inspected for damage to their electrical cords and buildup of dust (which can block airflow).

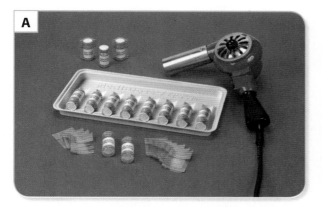
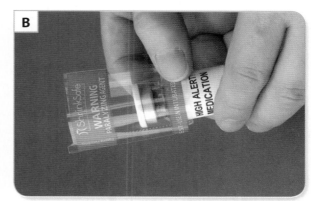
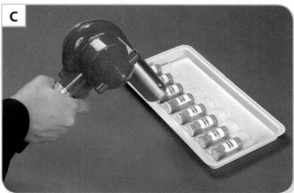
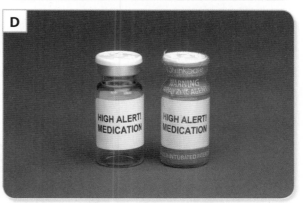

Figure 4-12 Heat gun and shrink wraps. (A) Shrink wrap system (B) Place the band over the vial (C) Use the heat gun to shrink the wrap to the vials (D) Vial before and after sealing with shrink wrap. (Courtesy of Medi-Dose, Inc./EPS, Inc., Ivyland, Pennsylvania.)

HOMOGENIZERS

Homogenizers are used to reduce particle size, usually for injectable products where particle size is essential. They are basically made up of a high-speed turbine that is mounted to a series of blades that rotate at

multiple angles (Figure 4-13). The blades of a homogenizer are first sterilize
in an autoclave, then lowered into a beaker of the desired solution and ru
at very high speeds. The solution is collected on the blade and shot out o
a very small hole in the shaft of the homogenizer assembly. After use, th
homogenizer can be wiped with isopropyl alcohol, but the blades shoul
also be re-sterilized in an autoclave. Homogenizers should be maintained b
an authorized service company.

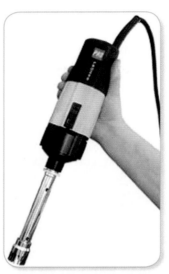

Figure 4-13 Homogenizer. (Courtesy of Lab Depot, Inc.,
Dawsonville, Georgia.)

HOT PLATES

Hot plates are used for fast heating of substances and are available wit
ceramic or aluminum tops, which heat to different temperature levels (th
ceramic tops heat to higher temperatures). Hot plates resemble weigh
scales, with a flat surface that conducts heat and a front panel with control
and a temperature display (Figure 4-14). They feature digital warnin

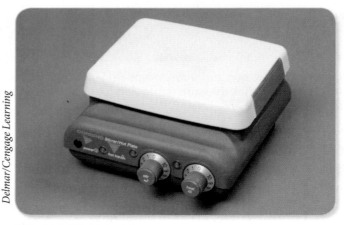

Delmar/Cengage Learning

Figure 4-14 Hot plate.

systems, digital settings, and high-wattage heating elements, and may even be available with microprocessors that offer automated stirring. Commonly used hot plates are of the low-temperature variety (25 to 120°C). After completely cooling, hot plates may be wiped with isopropyl alcohol for easy cleaning. It is important to check their electrical cords for potential damage that could result in a fire.

DRYING OVENS

Drying ovens usually contain several racks that are housed in steel panels bearing a plasticized exterior coating. They are ideal for general laboratory drying, sterilization (including equipment and some supplies), stress testing, moisture analysis, and curing. They are available in many different sizes and usually feature electronic controls with different-colored lights that signify which portion of their cycle they are in. Drying ovens may be easily cleaned with alcohol or detergents, but should be maintained by an authorized service company.

DRYING RACKS

Drying racks include stainless steel pegboards and glassware drying racks. They offer drip troughs, catch drains, interchangeable pegs, and the capacity to be autoclaved for sterilization. Drying racks may be easily cleaned with alcohol or detergents.

HEAT SEALERS

Heat sealers are ideal for preparing samples of flexible packaging materials. Some are digital in design and provide control over sealing pressure, temperature, automatic sample loading, and processing time. Heat sealers allow packages of different types to be securely sealed without damage to the chemicals, drugs, or other substances they may contain. Heat sealers generally require little cleaning, usually with mild detergents, but should be maintained by an authorized service company.

DRY BATHS

Dry baths may be available that either chill or heat samples (or both). The dry baths that both chill and heat are commonly available with temperature ranges of as low as −10 to 100 °C. Some dry baths also offer variable-speed orbital mixing while chilling or heating is occurring. Dry baths may be easily cleaned with alcohol or detergents, but should be maintained by an authorized service company.

BRUSHES

A broad range of medical brushes are used for sampling, cleaning, an microbrushing. Brushes may be made from natural or synthetic bristl materials. They may be designed for microbiology, cytology, and man other areas of medicine. Brushes may be soaked and cleaned with alcohol o detergents.

TONGS

Laboratory tongs include crucible tongs with or without ridges, beake tongs, flask tongs, and test tube holders (Figure 4-15). They are used for th sterile grasping and maneuvering of a variety of different types of laborator equipment. Tongs can be easily cleaned with alcohol or detergents, and ma be autoclaved.

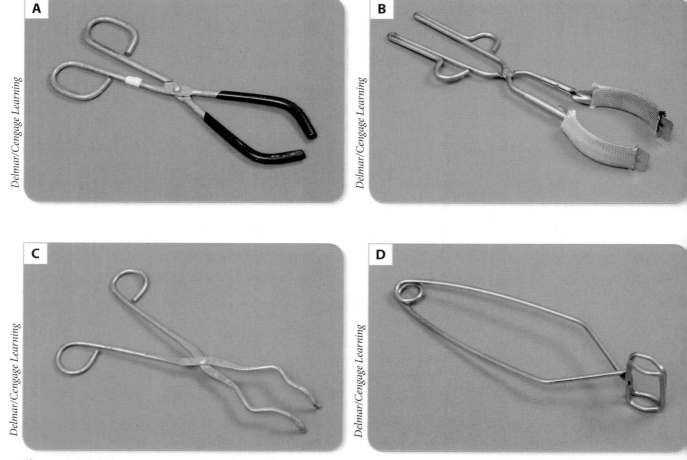

Figure 4-15 Laboratory tongs. (A and B) Beaker tongs (C) Crucible tongs (D) Test tube holder.

CRIMPERS

Crimpers are primarily used to seal vials and other containers with caps (Figure 4-16). Crimpers may also be used for pneumatic equipment and other activities. Some crimpers are designed for use with robotic machinery. Stainless steel vial crimpers are capable of withstanding aggressive sterilization and cleaning techniques. Usually, crimpers and related equipment such as decrimpers (also known as *decappers*) are used in pharmacies that solely handle extemporaneous compounding. Crimpers may be easily cleaned with alcohol or detergents and may be autoclaved.

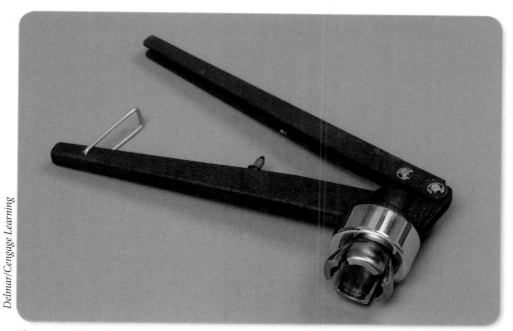

Delmar/Cengage Learning

Figure 4-16 Crimpers.

Procedure: Crimping Vials

Objective: To properly use a crimper to cap a vial.

Equipment Needed: crimper, vial, cap.

Step 1: Using proper clean technique, place the rubber stop on the vial (Figure 4-17A).

Step 2: Place the metal cap over the stoppered vial or bottle (Figure 4-17B).

Step 3: Adjust the pressure block in the crimper head according the manufacturer's instructions, using the supplied Allen wrench (this adjusts the length of stroke that occurs when pressure is applied).

Step 4: Place the crimper over the cap and squeeze according to the manufacturer's instructions (Figure 4-17C).

Step 5: Inspect the vial or bottle to be sure that the cap is properly sealed and crimped (Figure 4-17D).

Procedure: *(Continued)*

Figure 4-17 Use of a crimper. (A) Place the rubber stopper on the bottle (B) Place the cap on the stoppered bottle (C) Place the crimper over cap and squeeze (D) Inspect the cap on the bottle.

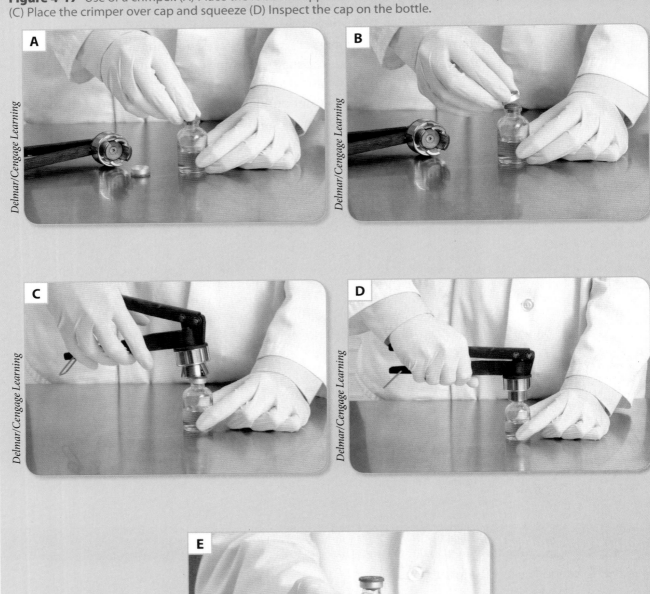

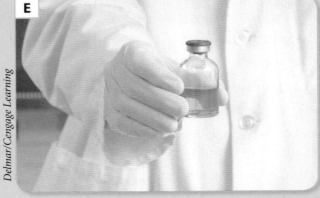

DECAPPERS

Decappers are also known as "decrimpers." Their uses are similar to the uses of crimpers, and they can also be used in robotics. They are also usually made of stainless steel, and allow aggressive sterilization and cleaning techniques. Decappers may be easily cleaned with alcohol or detergents, and may be autoclaved.

Procedure : Decapping Vials

Objective: To properly decap a vial using the proper tools.

Equipment Needed: decapper, vial.

Step 1: Place the decapper over the cap of the vial or bottle (Figure 4-18A).

Step 2: Squeeze the cap with the decapper.

Step 3: Twist the cap off (Figure 4-18B).

Step 4: Make sure to use clean technique so as not to contaminate the vial or bottle.

Figure 4-18 Use of a decrimper. (A) Place device over cap (B) Squeeze and twist cap off.

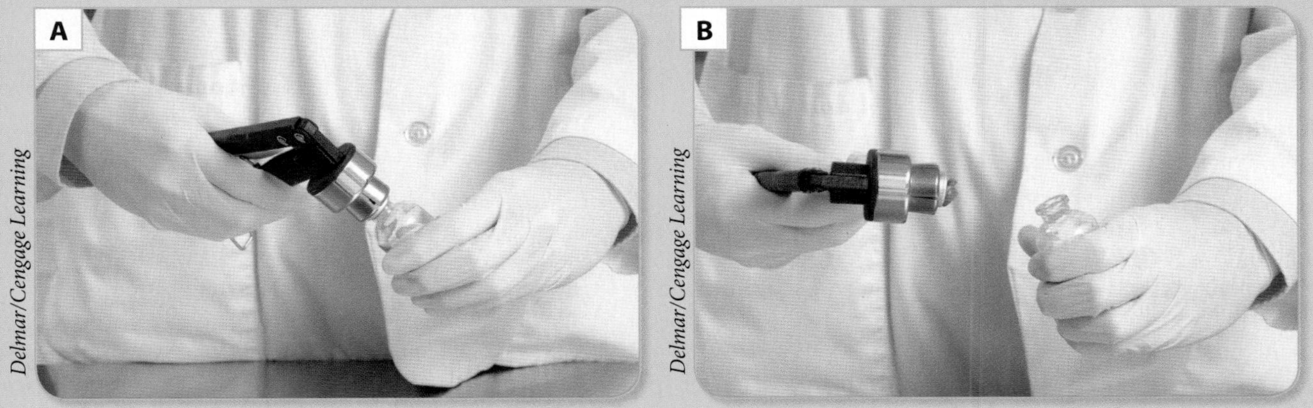

Delmar/Cengage Learning

SUPPOSITORY MOLDS

Suppository molds may be made of aluminum, plastic, flexible rubber, or very hard rubber (Figure 4-19). The aluminum suppository molds commonly range from 1 g to 2.5 g in size and are held together with nuts or a centered screw. Plastic suppository shells come in long strips, are disposable, and are heat-sealed once the desired mixture has been poured and hardened. Flexible rubber suppository molds are ideal if suppositories need to be refrigerated the finished suppositories may be "pushed" out of each cavity once they have congealed. Molds that are made of very hard rubber are held together by screws, and the suppositories they contain may be difficult to remove if they are too soft in their final form. If more than one suppository mold is used during compounding, the mold halves must not be mixed up, because they are specific to each other. When cleaning, they must be handled carefully to avoid creating scratches or grooves. Damage of this type can change the concentration of the completed suppository and also make them difficult to remove from the mold without breaking or cracking. Reusable suppository molds may be easily cleaned with alcohol or detergents.

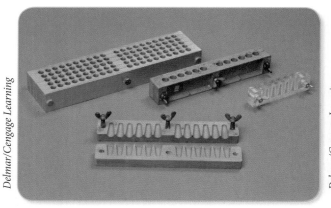
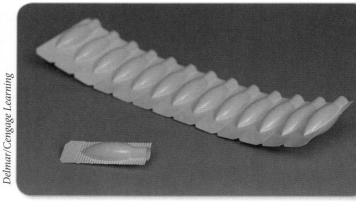

Delmar/Cengage Learning

Figure 4-19 Suppository molds.

ULTRASONIC CLEANERS

Ultrasonic cleaners are also known as *ultrasonic baths* and can clean metal and plastic equipment (Figure 4-20). They effectively remove blood, proteins, contaminants, grease, waxes, and oils. They work by moving sound waves through a heated solution to create **cavitation**, which is the rapid swelling and collapsing of microscopic bubbles. Advantages of ultrasonic cleaners are:

- Faster, safer, and more thorough than other clearing methods.
- Powerful enough to remove heavy oils.
- Consistent enough to manage difficult lab cleanups.
- Safe enough for delicate electronic components.
- Designed to be functional, reliable, and easy to use.

Ultrasonic cleaners may be easily cleaned with alcohol or detergents, but they should be maintained by an authorized service company.

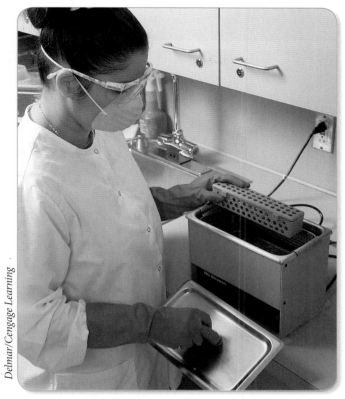

Delmar/Cengage Learning

Figure 4-20 Ultrasonic cleaning unit.

Procedure: *Use of an Ultrasonic Cleaner*

Objective: To properly use an ultrasonic cleaner to clean contaminated instruments.

Equipment Needed: ultrasonic cleaner, instruments, solvent.

Step 1: Fill the cleaning chamber with the appropriate solvent (most commonly, de-ionized water or isopropyl alcohol).

Step 2: Place the instrument to be cleaned within the cleaning chamber, making sure it is completely covered by the solvent.

Step 3: Turn the ultrasonic cleaner on and set it according to the instructions of the unit.

Step 4: Make sure the cleaning process lasts for the exact required time.

Step 5: Turn off the cleaner and remove the cleaned instrument using sterile equipment and technique.

Step 6: Clean the ultrasonic cleaning chamber using the manufacturer's guidelines.

PIPETTES AND PIPETTE FILLERS

Pipettes are used to measure small amounts of solution very accurately using a bulb (a pipette filler) to draw solution into the pipette (Figure 4-21A). Pipettes are durable and easy to clean. Pipette fillers are commonly made

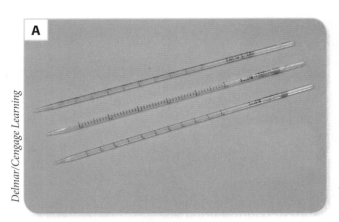

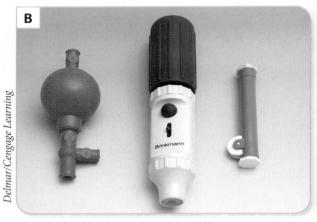

Figure 4-21 (A) Pipette (B) Pipetting aids.

of rubber with stainless steel valves (Figure 4-21B). They do away with the hazardous practice of pipetting by mouth, which is never recommended. Pipette fillers are very simple to use and offer the advantage of fitting with all sizes of pipettes, making them a must for every laboratory. Pipettes and pipette fillers are usually cleaned with de-ionized water, detergents, or isopropyl alcohol.

Procedure: Use of a Pipette

Objective: To properly and safely use a pipette to transfer liquids.

Equipment Needed: pipette, pipette filler, liquid, empty container.

Transfer the following amounts: ¼ of the pipette, ½ of the pipette, and a full pipette.

Step 1: Insert the pipette into the liquid to be withdrawn (Figure 4-22A).

Step 2: Squeeze the pipette's bulb (Figure 4-22B).

Step 3: Slowly release your grip until the desired amount is withdrawn (Figure 4-22C).

Step 4: Remove the pipette from the liquid and hold it above the container to which the liquid is being transferred.

Step 5: Remove the bulb holding your finger over the top of the pipette, slowly allowing the desired amount of liquid to flow into the container by releasing your finger from the top of the pipette (Figure 4-22D). You may also continue to use the bulb and squeeze the bulb to release the fluid in the pipette into the container.

Procedure: (Continued)

Figure 4-22 Use of a pipette. (A) Insert pipette into liquid (B) Squeeze the bulb (C) Release grip on the bulb until desired amount of liquid is in pipette (D) Release liquid into container.

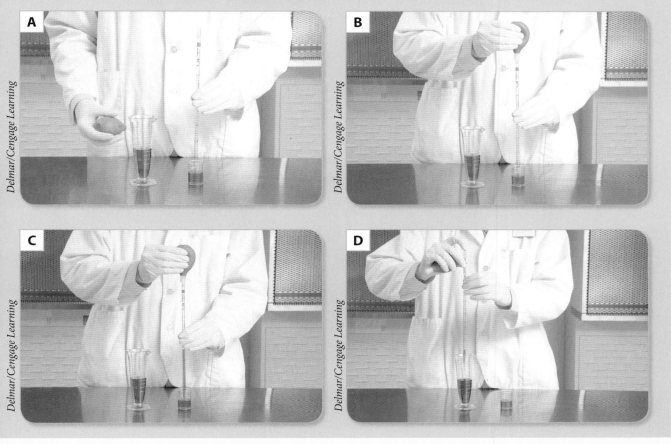

SPRAY BOTTLES

Laboratory spray bottles may be adjustable, be single- or double-headed, and offer virtually unbreakable sprayers. They are commonly used in the laboratory to rinse off glassware, filters, tubes, and other equipment. They can vary the flows of solutions they contain, even producing a fine mist if desired. Spray bottles may be easily rinsed and cleaned with detergents.

GLASS STIRRING RODS

Stirring rods may be made of glass, rubber, polypropylene, or bendable Teflon®, and are used to stir a variety of solutions or mixtures in the laboratory (Figure 4-23). Glass stirring rods usually have polished, rounded ends, and may have rubber sleeves fit over their tips. Polypropylene stirring rods have a flattened end that may also be used as a scoop or small spatula. Teflon stirring rods are flexible yet unbreakable, containing a wire insert that bends to any shape. Stirring rods are easily cleaned by isopropyl alcohol or detergents. Glass stirring rods should be checked for chips or cracks prior to use and discarded if they are visibly damaged.

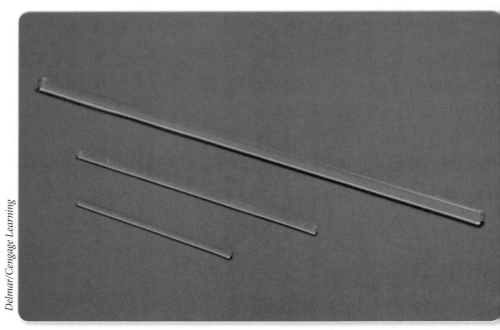

Delmar/Cengage Learning

Figure 4-23   Stirring rods.

GRADUATES

To measure liquids, conical or cylindrical graduates may be used. **Conical graduates** have wide tops and thinner bases, tapering from the top to the bottom (Figure 4-24A). They are easier to clean than cylindrical graduates. **Cylindrical graduates** are designed with a narrow diameter that is the same from top to base. Cylindrical graduates are more accurate than conical graduates (see Figure 4-24B). Graduates may be easily cleaned with alcohol or detergents.

These types of graduates are generally calibrated in metric units (cubic centimeters) while conical graduates are usually calibrated in both metric and apothecary units. Glass graduates are handy for accurate measurements of small volumes of liquids and will not cloud if exposed to materials such as hydrocarbons.

The proper technique of calculating the volume of a liquid in a graduate is by reading the **meniscus**. The meniscus is the bottom portion of the concave surface of a liquid. This shape is achieved because of the surface

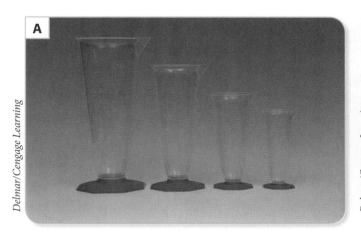

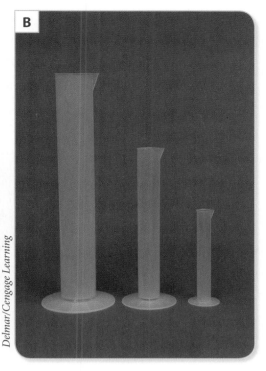

Figure 4-24 (A) Conical graduates (B) Cylindrical graduates.

tension of the liquid. The meniscus is used to measure the volume of a liquid in a container, such as a graduate. With most liquids, the meniscus curves upward near the sides of the container, making the center of the curve of the meniscus appear lower than the sides. It is this point, the lowest part of this curve, that should be used to determine the amount of liquid in the container (Figure 4-25).

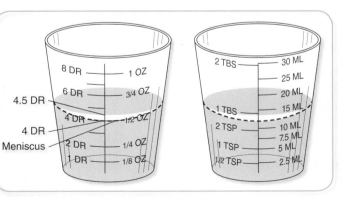

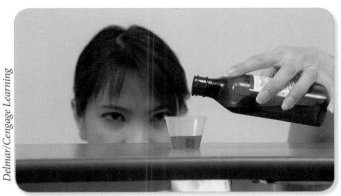

Figure 4-25 Reading the meniscus.

For accuracy, the smallest available graduate should always be used to measure a certain volume of liquid. Avoid measuring volumes that are less than 20 percent of the graduate's capacity because the accuracy would not be acceptable. Both conical and cylindrical graduates have graduated markings for measuring specific fluid volumes.

Exercise

Objective: To become familiar reading liquid measurements.

Look at each of the figures and write the reading at the meniscus.

A. _____

B. _____

C. _____

D. _____

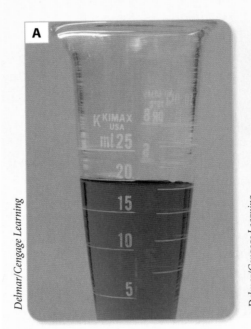

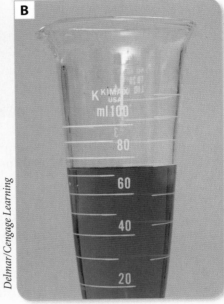

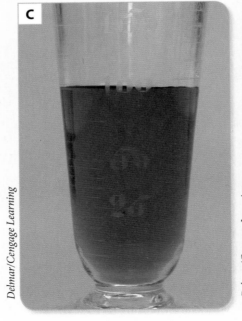

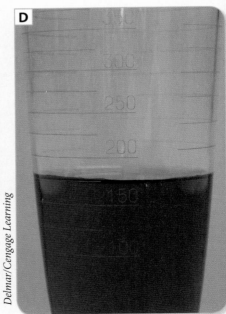

Delmar/Cengage Learning

DROPPERS

Droppers are used to deliver small doses of liquid medication (Figure 4-26). They are calibrated to select the amount of liquid substance that is to be administered. Droppers are especially useful for administering medications to infants and children. Droppers may be easily cleaned with alcohol or detergents.

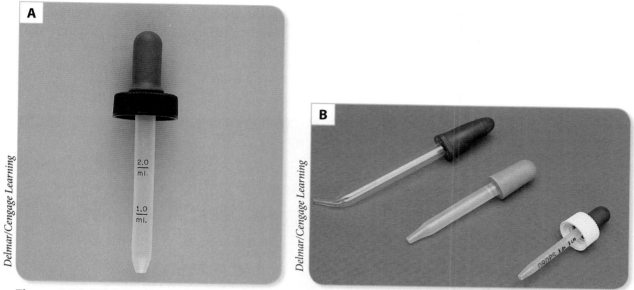

Delmar/Cengage Learning

Figure 4-26 (A) Calibrated dropper (B) Glass, plastic, and calibrated droppers.

Exercise

Objective: To become familiar with the calibrations of droppers.

Using the depictions of the three droppers below, mark the following three amounts of medications: 0.75 mL, 1 mL, and 1.5 mL.

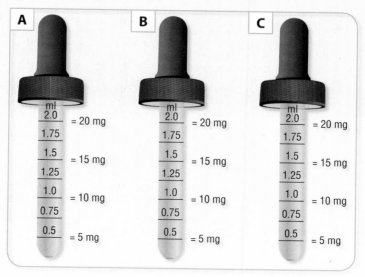

BEAKERS

Beakers are simple liquid containers that are usually cylindrical in shape, with a flat bottom. In the pharmacy, they commonly range in size from 25 mL to 600 mL. They may be made of glass, Pyrex®, plastic, Teflon, or other corrosion resistant materials (Figure 4-27). Beakers can be covered to prevent contamination or content loss, and may be graduated with various volume measurements on the sides. Beakers are distinguished from flasks in that their sides are straight rather than sloping. Beakers may be easily cleaned with alcohol or detergents.

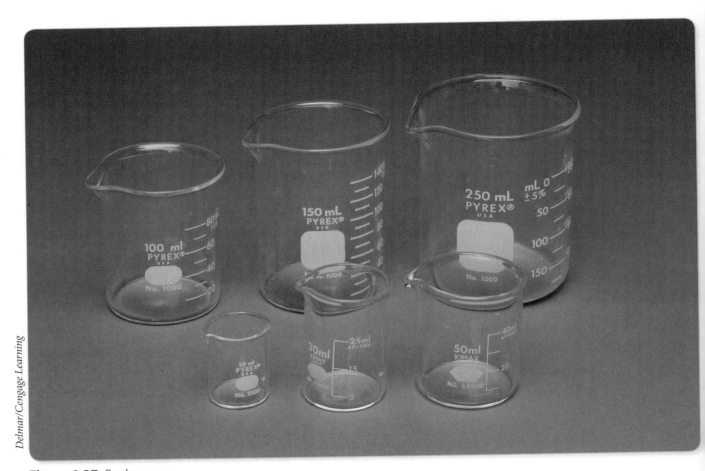

Figure 4-27 Beakers.

Beakers should not be used for measuring volumes because the are not as accurate as graduates. Beakers should be used to mix and mel substances.

BEAKER TONGS

Beaker tongs may have two or three *jaws*, and are usually made of stainless steel, or may be nickel-plated (Figure 4-28). They can handle various sizes of beakers (usually ranging from 50 to 2,000 mL in size). They are often resistant to corrosion and may offer jaws made of fiberglass. Beaker tongs may be easily cleaned with alcohol or detergents, and may be autoclaved.

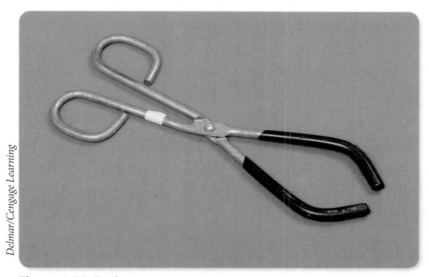

Delmar/Cengage Learning

Figure 4-28 Beaker tongs.

Exercise

Objective: To become familiar with the proper use of beaker tongs.

Practice pouring liquids into beakers and transferring them for heating by using beaker tongs and placing them onto a hot plate.

FUNNELS

Funnels are tubes that have a wide mouth and a narrow bottom (Figure 4-29). They are used when pouring liquids from one container into another, commonly in conjunction with filter papers in order to remove insoluble particles or contaminants. They look like a hollow cone with a slim tube or pipe extending from the narrowest point. They are used for conveying liquid substances downward. Funnels may be easily cleaned with alcohol or detergents.

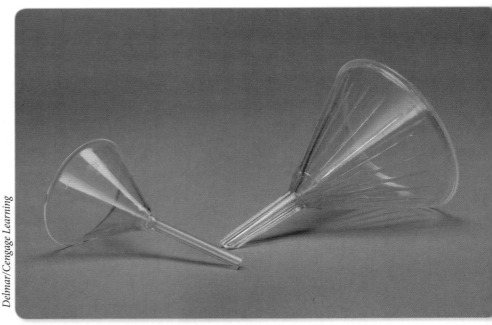

Delmar/Cengage Learning

Figure 4-29 Funnels.

CAPSULE-FILLING EQUIPMENT

Capsule-filling equipment today is more accurate and efficient tha ever before. A wide variety of automated machinery in many different size is available that can fill more than 12,000 capsules per hour. These type of machines are not intended for use in small-volume retail or hospita pharmacies. Manual capsule-filling systems are still used, usually for 100 t 300 capsules at a time. Empty capsule shells commonly range in size from 5 to 000. Capsule-filling machinery and equipment may be easily cleane with alcohol or detergents, but should be maintained by an authorize service company.

TABLET MOLDS

Molded tablets are usually made by mixing active drugs with sugar or other diluents that are water-soluble and don't degrade the tablet effectiveness. Lactose and mannitol are the preferred diluents. Tablet triturat molds are made of metal, with plate cavity sizes ranging between 60 mg an 100 mg. Molded tablets are compounded by preparing a powder mixtur which is then sifted and moistened (usually using a mixture of water an alcohol). The mixture is then pressed into the tablet cavities with sufficier pressure to form them, then forced out of the cavities and allowed to dr Tablet molds may be easily cleaned with alcohol or detergents.

CARTS

Carts are heavy two-wheeled vehicles, commonly without springs, for the conveyance of heavy goods. Pharmacy carts are used to transport and/or store medications (Figure 4-30). Many carts feature vinyl bumpers and bottom outriggers that guide carts away from walls. Carts can be easily cleaned with isopropyl alcohol or detergents.

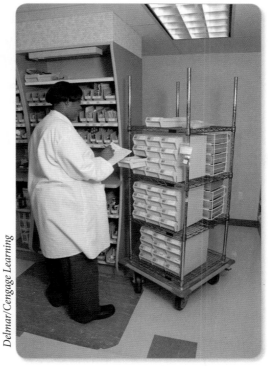

Delmar/Cengage Learning

Figure 4-30 Medication carts.

REFRIGERATORS AND FREEZERS

Pharmacy refrigerators and freezers offer wide ranges of temperature control, bacteria-resistant coatings, and self-closing door systems (see Figure 4-31). Other models offer programmable defrost times, digital controls, and alarm/monitor systems. Refrigerators and freezers must have accurate thermometers, checked at least once per day to ensure proper temperature regulation. Refrigerators and freezers may be easily cleaned with isopropyl alcohol or detergents. They should be regularly checked to make sure that electrical cords are in good condition, door seals are working correctly, and air filters are clean and dust-free. Full maintenance of refrigerators and freezers should be performed by an authorized service company.

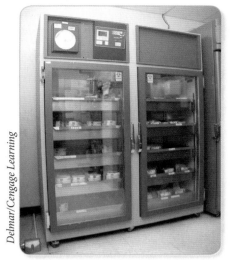

Delmar/Cengage Learning

Figure 4-31 Laboratory refrigerator.

SAFETY GLASSES, GLOVES, AND MASKS

Safety glasses, gloves, and masks are all used in the compounding pharmac[y] setting to enhance disease control and to prevent the transfer of pathogens t[o] and from the staff (Figure 4-32). They also protect technicians from exposur[e] to hazardous or potentially hazardous materials. Safety glasses generall[y] provide full frames with side shields to provide as much eye protection a[s] possible. Most gloves offer beaded cuffs for ease of use and ambidextrou[s] shapes that fit both hands. Most masks meet requirements for tuberculosis an[d] other airborne pathogen exposure control. Safety glasses may be easily cleane[d] with alcohol or detergents. Though there are washable cloth masks, the mo[st] common masks used today are disposable and intended for single use. Mo[st] gloves are designed for single use and are therefore also disposable.

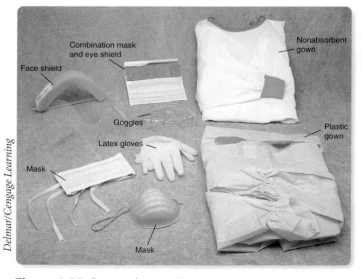

Delmar/Cengage Learning

Figure 4-32 Personal protective equipment.

SUMMARY

Pharmacy technicians are required to be familiar with various types of equipment and supplies that are needed for compounding drugs. Some state boards of pharmacy require specific minimum lists of equipment for compounding prescriptions. Each pharmacy is required to have a Class A prescription balance and/or an electronic balance. Compounding slabs (or ointment slabs) are flat glass surfaces used for mixing compounds. The most common equipment used for compounding includes: mortars, pestles, hot plates, forceps, suppository molds, graduates, beakers, and safety equipment such as glasses, gloves, and masks. Most vessels that are used to contain mixtures are marked with graduated measurements.

REVIEW QUESTIONS

Fill in the Blank

1. Weights made from corrosion-resistant metals, such as _____, are preferred.

2. Mortars are available in glass, Wedgwood, and _____.

3. Glass mortars are preferred for mixing _____ and _____ dosage forms.

4. Homogenizers are used to reduce _____ size.

5. Aluminum suppository molds commonly range from 1 g to _____ g in size and are held together with nuts or a centered screw.

6. Ultrasonic cleaners are also known as ultrasonic _____ and can clean metal and plastic equipment.

7. _____ graduates are more accurate than _____ graduates.

8. Beakers are distinguished from flasks in that their sides are _____ rather than _____.

9. Spatulas are available in stainless steel, _____, or _____.

10. A counter balance is capable of weighing larger quantities, up to about _____ kg.

Matching

1. _____ Used to mix compounds on an ointment slabs.

2. _____ May offer jaws made of fiberglass.

3. _____ Are the same from top to base.

4. _____ Used for measuring bulk products.

5. _____ Used to shrink bands onto vials.

6. _____ Also called ointment slabs.

    A. Compounding slabs
    B. Heat guns
    C. Cylindrical graduates
    D. Beaker tongs
    E. Counter balances
    F. Spatulas

OBJECTIVES

Upon completion of this chapter, the student should be able to:

1. Demonstrate the compounding of an ointment.
2. Demonstrate the compounding of a capsule.
3. Demonstrate the compounding of a suppository.
4. Demonstrate the compounding of a hand cream.
5. Demonstrate the compounding of a suspension.
6. Define the terms "ointment," "paste," and "suppository."

GLOSSARY

Bulk compounding formula record – Listing of ingredients and recipe for a specific medication formulation; also known as a master formula sheet.

Capsule – A solid dosage form featuring a drug contained inside an external shell.

Creams – Pharmaceutical preparations that combine oil with water, and are usually used topically.

Elixirs – Liquid dosage forms that are sweetened, and contain alcohol and water.

Emulsion – A type of suspension that consists of two different liquids and an emulsifying agent (an *emulsifier*) that holds them together.

Gel – A jellylike substance commonly used for topical application that consists of particles mixed into a liquid, usually with an absorption base.

Geometric dilution – The mixing of a medication with an equal weight of a diluent, then an equivalent amount of diluent, until all the diluent is mixed in.

Insufflation – A powdered medication blown into a nasal passage or ear canal.

Levigate – To grind a powder into a smooth surface using moisture.

Liquid drugs – The most common form of compounded medications.

Magmas – Gels that have large particle sizes in a two-phase system.

Master formula sheet – Listing of ingredients and recipe for a specific medication formulation; also known as a bulk compounding formula record.

Ointment – A highly viscous or semisolid substance used on the skin that may be referred to as an *emollient* or a *salve*.

Paste – A semisolid pharmaceutical preparation that is intended for external use.

Powder – A dosage form that may be used when a drug's stability or solubility is a concern; they are often mixed into foods or liquids.

Solution – A liquid dosage form containing active ingredients that are dissolved in a liquid solvent.

Solvent – A liquid vehicle used to dissolve active ingredients in a solution.

Suppositories – Semisolid dosage forms that may be inserted into the rectum, vagina, or urethra for localized or systemic effects.

Suspension – A liquid dosage form that contains solid drug particles floating in a liquid medium which are easy to compound, but physically unstable; suspensions must be shaken well before they are administered.

Tablet – A solid dosage form that is made by compressing the powdered form of a drug and bulk filling material under high pressure.

Triturated – Reduced to a fine powder by grinding.

OVERVIEW

Most of the time, pharmaceutical manufacturers provide what patients need, and do an excellent job. These manufacturers have invested money and effort into research and development for their products. Extemporaneous compounding by pharmacists and technicians meets the additional needs of patients that traditionally manufactured pharmaceutical products do not meet.

The need for compounding training and experience is addressed by short courses, continuing education, increased curriculums, and apprenticeships. Additional training areas are required to provide the experience that is needed for compounding prescriptions accurately and safely.

Only properly educated and fully trained pharmacy technicians should be involved in pharmaceutical compounding. When technicians are required to compound drug products, but do not possess the required techniques or skills, they should participate in continuing professional education programs that have been designed to give them proper training. These programs may address the scientific basis, practical skills, and new technologies with which pharmacy technicians must be familiar in order to be able to accurately compound various drugs, agents, and substances.

In the pharmacy, a **master formula sheet** is commonly used to list all the ingredients required to compound a specific formulation. It lists the amounts of each ingredient to be used, manufacturer, lot number, and expiration date, and has a section that the personnel who compound and check the mixture can initial. It also lists the actual procedure to be followed for compounding. Often, these sheets are printed on card stock, which is heavier than normal paper. Master formula sheets are also referred to as **bulk compounding formula records**. See Figure 5-1 for a sample master formula sheet.

MASTER FORMULA SHEET – NON-STERILE MANUFACTURING

PRODUCT: **HYDROCHLOROTHIAZIDE** 5 mg/mL AND **SPIRONOLACTONE** 5 mg/mL SUSPENSION

Date Prepared: ____________________ **FINAL PRODUCT CHECKED BY:** ____________________

EXPIRY DATE: ____________________

INGREDIENT	MANUFACTURER	LOT #	MAN. EXPIRY DATE	FORMULA QUANTITY	QUANTITY USED	MFG BY	CHK BY
Hydrochlorothiazide 25 mg Spironolactone 25 mg tablet				20			
Ora-Blend®	Paddock			qs to 100 ML			

EQUIPMENT
- Mortar and pestle
- Graduated Cylinder

MANUFACTURING DIRECTIONS
1. Crush tablets to make a fine powder in a mortar.
2. Levigate powder with a small amount of the vehicle to make a fine paste.
3. Continue to add vehicle until product liquid enough to transfer to a graduated cylinder.
4. Rinse mortar several times with vehicle and add to product in graduated cylinder.
5. QS to final volume with vehicle.
6. Dispense in amber plastic bottles. May be refrigerated or stored at room temperature.

FINAL APPEARANCE

Opaque white suspension

SAMPLE LABEL

HYDROCHLOROTHIZIADE 5 mg/mL
and SPIRONOLACTONE 5 mg/mL Suspension
Shake well. Refrigerate. Take with Food.
Date Prepared: Date Expired:

STABILITY
60 days in fridge or at room temperature.

REFERENCE(S)
- Nahata MC, Hipple TF, Pediatric Drug Formulations, 4th ed. 2000, pp 115
- Allen LV, Erickson MA. AJHP 1996, 53: 2304-9

MASTER Sheet Revision Dates: ____________________ ***Final Approval By:***

The non-sterile manufacturing formulas are provided for informational purposes for qualified health care professionals. The hospital will not assume responsibility for the continued currency of the information, any errors or ommissions, and/or any consequences arising from the use of the information outside of CHEO.

Figure 5-1 Master formula sheet.

COMPOUNDING OF SOLID DRUGS

The most common dosage forms of solid drugs include tablets, capsules and powders.

Tablets

A **tablet** is a solid dosage form that is made by compressing the powdered form of a drug and bulk filling material under high pressure. While most tablets are shaped like cylinders, they may be in different shapes. Caplets, for example, are tablets that are stamped into a capsule shape. Tablets may or may not have special coatings or colorings. Special molds consisting of pegboards and perforated plates are used when manufacturing tablets. Diluents that are used in this type of compounding are usually mixtures of lactose, sucrose, and a moistening agent (usually ethyl alcohol mixed with water). The diluent is triturated with the active ingredients, making a paste with the moistening agent. This is spread into the mold, with the tablets then punched out and allowed to dry.

Procedure: Compounding Tablets

Objective: To understand how to properly compound tablets.

Equipment Needed: tablet mold, base material, balance, active ingredients, alcohol and distilled water mixture, compounding slab, rubber spatula, airtight container, label.

Tablets may be easily compounded with the following steps:

Step 1: Gather all equipment and supplies that are required.

Step 2: Make sure that the tablet mold has been calibrated so that the desired weight of each individual tablet will be achieved; to do this, you must:

- Prepare a batch of the base material that will be used in the final tablets.
- Fill 10 of the mold cavities to capacity.
- Let these test tablets set.
- Remove them from the mold.
- Weigh these test tablets.
- Divide by 10 to verify the weight of each tablet; it should be the weight desired for each of the final tablets.

Step 3: Combine the correct amount of active ingredient (Figure 5-2A) with a small amount of the tablet base (Figure 5-2B).

Step 4: Triturate the two ingredients (Figure 5-2C). Continue to add in the tablet base in small amounts and triturate with the active ingredient.

Step 5: Dampen the mixture with a mixture of 50 to 80 percent alcohol and distilled water (Figure 5-2D).

Procedure: (Continued)

Step 6: Triturate until the mixture has a dough-like consistency; it should be pliable (Figure 5-2E).

Step 7: Force the wet mixture into the holes in the top plate with a spatula, packing each cavity to capacity (Figure 5-2F).

Step 8: Working quickly to avoiding premature drying, smooth the top edges with the spatula and remove excess mixture (Figures 5-2G and 5-2H).

Step 9: Allow the tablets to dry partially.

Step 10: Remove the top plate, invert it, and align it to the bottom plate (Figures 5-2I through 5-2K).

Step 11: Gently press down to allow the pegs to push the tablets out of the holes, leaving the plates intact (Figure 5-2L).

Step 12: Allow the tablets to dry.

Step 13: After drying, carefully transfer the tablets to a porous material that will allow for good airflow to dry them thoroughly.

Step 14: Package the finished tablets into an airtight container (Figure 5-2M).

Step 15: Label with proper labeling (Figure 5-2N). The tablets are now ready for dispensing.

Figure 5-2 Compounding tablets. (A) Place the active ingredient into a mortar (B) Add in a small amount of base (C) Triturate the active ingredient with the base (D) Add alcohol and continue to triturate.

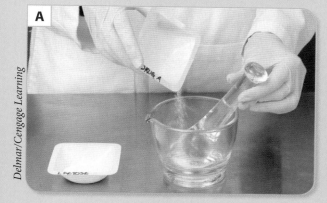
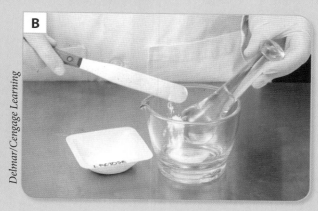
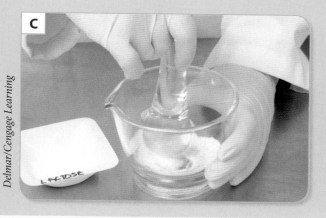
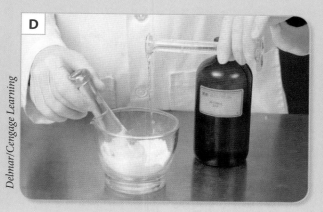

Procedure: (Continued)

Figure 5-2 Compounding tablets. (E) The material will form into a dough-like consistency (F) Force mixture into holes in mold (G and H) Scrape excess off the top of the mold (I and J) Remove the top plate and invert it.

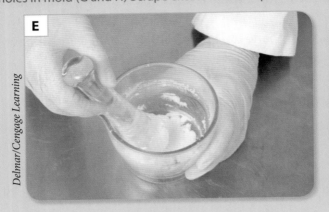

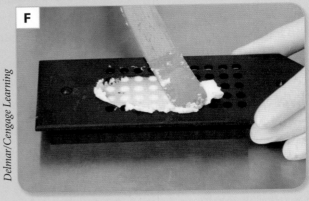

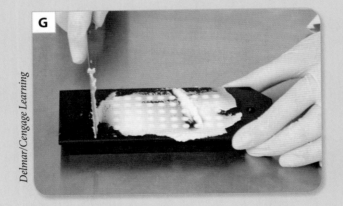

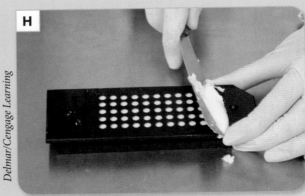

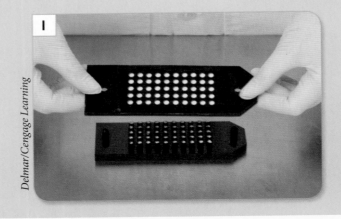

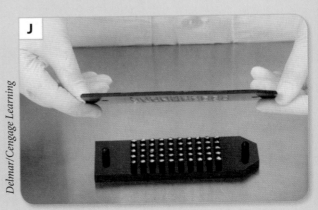

Procedure: (Continued)

Figure 5-2 Compounding tablets. (K) Align the top plate to the bottom plate (L) press the plate down to pop the pills out (M) Package tablets (N) Label package.

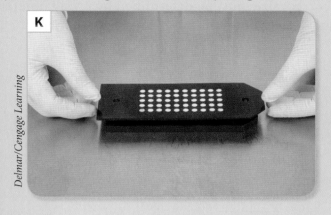

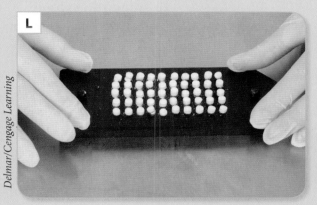

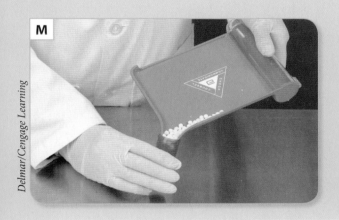

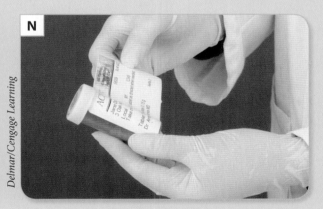

Exercise: Various capsule sizes

Objective: To identify various capsule sizes.

Select 10 different bottles of medication capsules and identify the largest versus the smallest.

Capsules

A **capsule** is a solid dosage form featuring a drug contained inside an external shell. Capsule shells are usually made of hard gelatin. They enclose or encapsulate powder or beads of medication. Soft gelatin capsules are used to contain drugs that exist in a liquid form. An example of this type of capsule is a soft gelatin vitamin E capsule.

Hard gelatin capsules may be manually filled during extemporaneous compounding. For human patients, capsule sizes range from number 5 (the smallest) to number 000 (the largest) (Figure 5-3). Usually, number 0 is the largest oral size capsule suitable for most patients. When preparing both hard and soft capsules, the correct size must be determined by trying different sizes, weighing them, and determining which is the most appropriate.

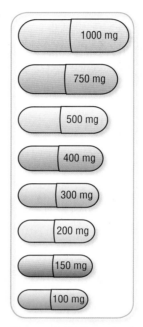

1000 mg

750 mg

500 mg

400 mg

300 mg

200 mg

150 mg

100 mg

Figure 5-3 Capsule sizes.

Procedure: Hand Filling of Capsules Using the Punch Method

Objective: To properly compound capsules.

Equipment Needed: capsule body, active ingredients, spatula, mortar and pestle, balance, bottle, label.

Step 1: Gather all equipment and supplies that are required (Figure 5-4A).

Step 2: Separate the body and cap of each capsule.

Step 3: Weigh the base material (Figure 5-4B).

Step 4: Grind the base material in a mortar and pestle (Figure 5-4C).

Step 5: Add the powdered active ingredients to the base material in the mortar and pestle.

Step 6: Press the empty capsule body repeatedly into the powder until full (Figure 5-4D).

Step 7: Push the other half of the capsule into the powder while slightly rotating the body of the capsule (Figure 5-4E).

Step 8: Weigh the capsule to ensure the accurate dose.

Procedure: (Continued)

Step 9: Place an empty capsule of the same size on one side of the balance pan to compare to the weight of the filled capsule; this determines the weight of the capsule shell. No more than 10 percent over or under the intended weight is acceptable.

Step 10: Wipe each capsule clean of any powder or oil and dispense in a suitable prescription vial.

Step 11: Label the medication.

For a large number of capsules, capsule-filling machines can be used to save time.

Figure 5-4 Compounding capsule by hand. (A) Gather equipment (B) Weigh ingredients (C) Grind ingredients.

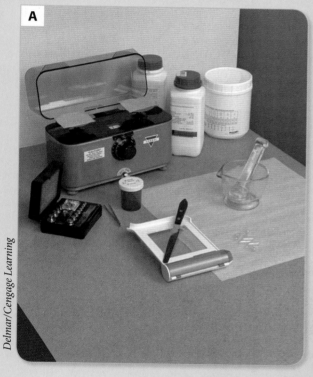

Delmar/Cengage Learning

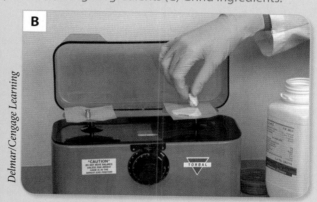

Delmar/Cengage Learning

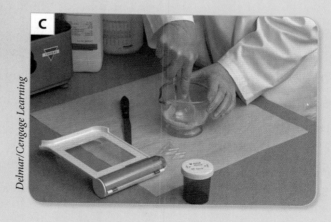

Delmar/Cengage Learning

Procedure: (Continued)

Figure 5-4 Compounding capsule by hand. (D) Fill capsule using punch method (E) Place cap on capsule.

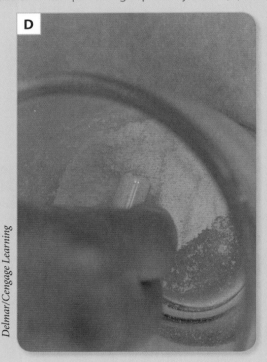

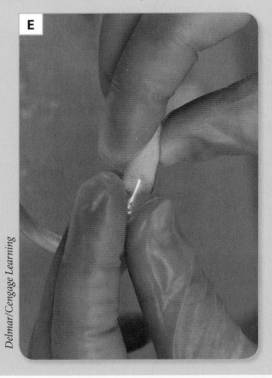

Delmar/Cengage Learning

Procedure: Machine Filling of Capsules

Objective: To properly operate and fill capsules using a capsule-filling machine.

Equipment Needed: capsule-filling machine, active ingredients, capsule body, balance, bottle, label.

Note: Machine filling of capsules involves a powder dam, which is clamped to the work surface to keep powder from falling over the edges of the surface.

Step 1: Gather all equipment and supplies that are required.

Step 2: Pour the empty capsules onto the orienter and shake back and forth to fill the slots (Figures 5-5A and 5-5B).

Step 3: Pour the leftover capsules back into the container (Figure 5-5C).

Step 4: Place the orienter on the filler locking plate at mark I (Figures 5-5D and 5-5E).

Step 5: Push the sliding portion of the orienter left to drop the capsules into the filler; when the orienter is removed, every other row will be filled (Figure 5-5F). Repeat steps 2 through 5, moving the orienter to mark II. When the orienter is removed, all slots will be filled (Figure 5-5G).

Step 6: Close the filler locking plate (Figure 5-5H) and slide the clamp to lock the bodies of the capsules into the filler (Figure 5-5I).

Step 7: Lift the top portion of filler by the handles to separate the capsule halves (Figure 5-5J).

Procedure: *(Continued)*

Step 8: Release the locking mechanism so that the capsule halves fall flush to the tray (Figure 5-5K).

Step 9: Place the powder tray on the filler (Figure 5-5L).

Step 10: Pour the powdered active ingredients over the empty capsule bases held by the machine (Figure 5-5M) and, using a wide spatula, sweep the powder into the capsule halves (Figure 5-5N). Continue to do this until the capsules are full (Figure 5-5O).

Step 11: Use a tamper to pack the capsules (Figures 5-5P and 5-5Q). Continue to use the spatula to fill in the capsules completely.

Step 12: Remove the powder tray and replace the top of the filler containing the tops of the capsules (Figure 5-5R).

Step 13: Squeeze the top and bottom plates together to combine the top and bottom halves of the capsules (Figures 5-5S and 5-5T).

Step 14: Open the top of the filler tray and remove the capsules, locking them together as you take them out of the filler tray (Figure 5-5U).

Step 15: Weigh finished capsules, checking for accuracy within 10 percent (as in hand filling). Record weights on a formula worksheet for proof of accuracy.

Step 16: Fill the bottle and label the medication.

Figure 5-5 Compounding capsules with capsule-filling machine. (A) Pour capsules in machine (B) Shake until capsules fall into slots (C) Discard excess capsules.

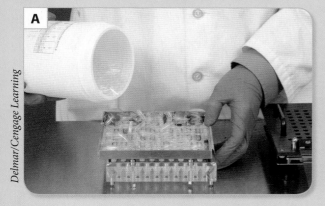

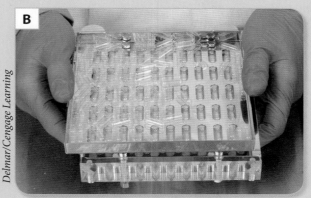

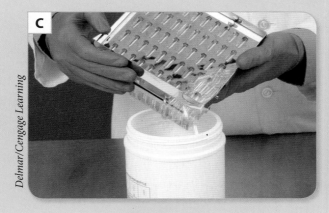

Procedure: (Continued)

Figure 5-5 Compounding capsules with capsule-filling machine. (D and E) Align tray with filler tray at slot I (F) Every other row should be filled with an empty capsule (G) Repeat aligning with slot II so that all rows are filled (H) Close the filler tray. (I) Lock it into place.

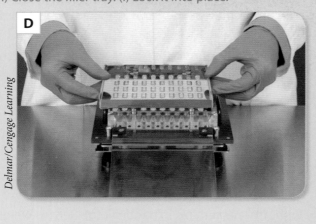

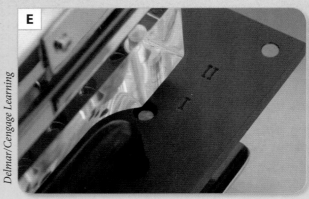

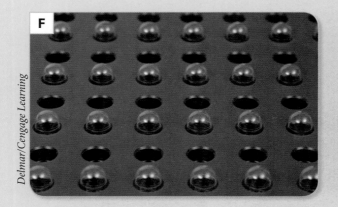

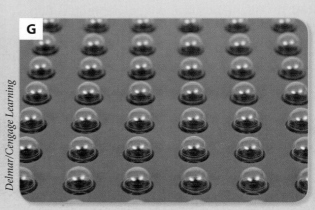

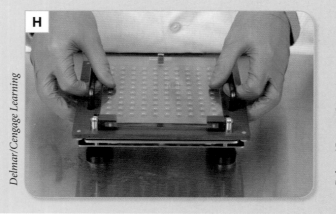

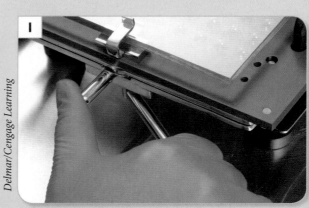

Procedure: (Continued)

Figure 5-5 Compounding capsules with capsule-filling machine. (J) Lift the top of filler tray to remove capsule tops (K) Release the lock so that capsule bottoms fall flush with tray (L) Place tray on top of filler tray (M) Add active ingredients (N and O) Use a spatula or tool to fill capsules.

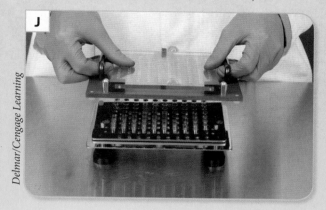

Delmar/Cengage Learning

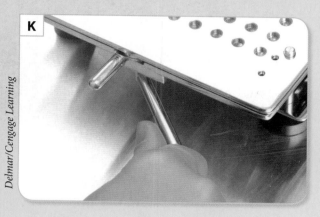

Delmar/Cengage Learning

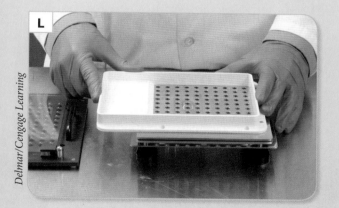

Delmar/Cengage Learning

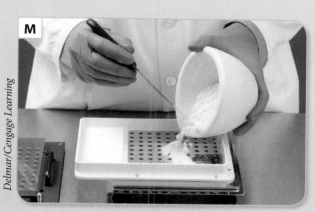

Delmar/Cengage Learning

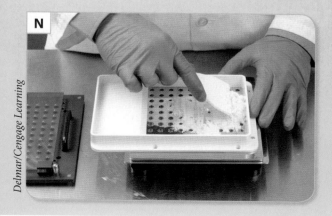

Delmar/Cengage Learning

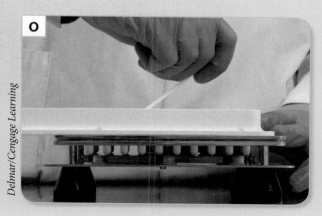

Delmar/Cengage Learning

Procedure: (Continued)

Figure 5-5 Compounding capsules with capsule-filling machine. (P and Q) Tamp down active ingredients (R) Once capsules are filled place top of filler tray on bottom portion (S and T) Squeeze the top and bottom together (U) Remove completed capsules and ensure they are locked.

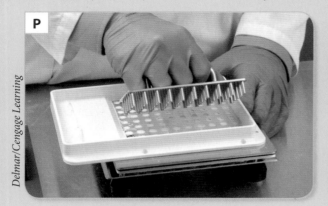

Delmar/Cengage Learning

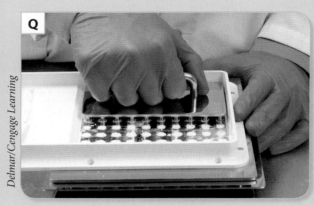

Delmar/Cengage Learning

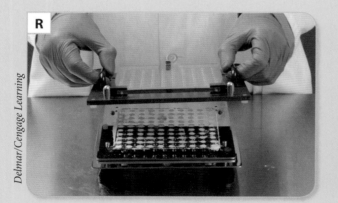

Delmar/Cengage Learning

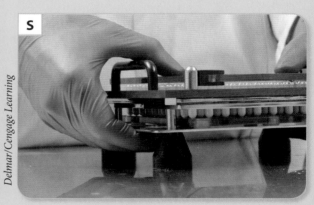

Delmar/Cengage Learning

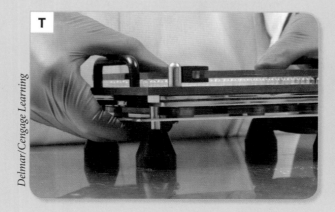

Delmar/Cengage Learning

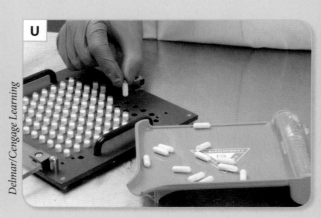

Delmar/Cengage Learning

Powders

When a drug's stability or solubility is a concern, powdered dosage forms may be used. They may be used either internally or externally. **Powders** are also used when patients would have difficulty in swallowing capsules, or when the powdered drug is too bulky to be made into capsules. Powders are often unpleasant in taste, and their use has declined. They are often mixed with food or liquids for ingestion. Inhaled powders are still commonly used to treat headaches. Sometimes, a process known as **insufflation** is used, wherein a powdered medication is blown into a nasal passage or an ear canal.

Powders may be blended using trituration (the creating of fine particles from a powder by grinding) in a mortar, stirred with a spatula, and sifted. If required, **geometric dilution** (the mixing of a medication with an equal weight of a diluent, then an equivalent amount of diluent, until all the diluent is mixed in) may be used. It is important to remember that when mixing heavier powders with lighter powders, the heavier powder should be placed on top of the lighter powder and then blended. When two or more powders are to be mixed, each powder should be pulverized separately to about the same particle size before they are blended.

Procedure: Compounding Powders

Objective: To properly prepare a compounded powder.

Equipment Needed: active ingredients, mortar and pestle, spatula, sieve, container, label.

Step 1: Gather all equipment and supplies that are required.

Step 2: Grind each powder in separate mortars to make the particle sizes as similar as possible.

Step 3: To begin mixing, start with the powder of smallest quantity (Figure 5-6A).

Step 4: Add the powder of next-smallest quantity, adding an identical quantity of this powder to the powder of smallest quantity so that the total quantity in this mortar is now doubled (Figure 5-6B).

Step 5: Triturate until blended (Figure 5-6C).

Step 6: Continue adding the powder in this same "doubling" manner (Figure 5-6D).

Step 7: Triturate until blended (Figure 5-6E).

Step 8: If there are additional powders to be blended, continue in the same manner until all the powders are combined.

Step 9: Triturate until all the powders are consistently blended.

Step 10: Stir the powders with a spatula.

Step 11: Sift the powders through a 100-size mesh sieve.

Step 12: Place the compounded powder into the proper container, or in the example of a headache powder, place individual doses into paper wrappers and fold them to contain the powders without spillage.

Step 13: Make sure to label the final package(s) or container(s) properly. The compounded powder is now ready to dispense to the patient.

Procedure: (Continued)

Figure 5-6 Compounding powders. (A) Place drug in mortar (B) Place an equal amount of powder in mortar with drug and triturate (C) Combine powders in mortar by doubling each time (D) Triturate.

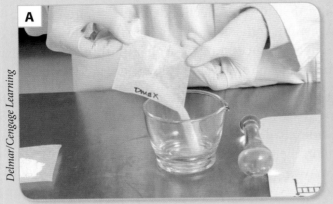

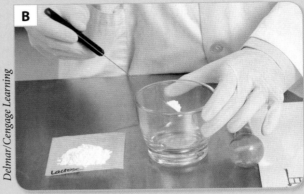

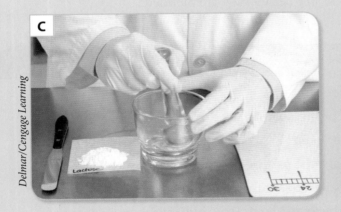

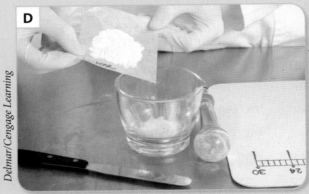

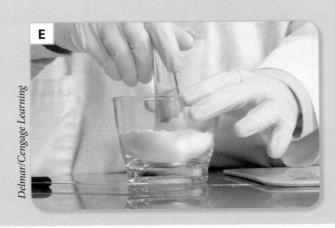

Exercise: Mixing powders

Objective: To understand the procedure required for mixing various quantities of powders.

Mix 5 grams of one powder with 2 grams of a different powder.

Lozenges

Lozenges are small medicated "candies" intended to be dissolved slowly within the mouth. They are also referred to as *troches*.

Procedure: Compounding Lozenges

Objective: To properly prepare compounded lozenges.

Equipment Needed: active ingredients, confectioner's sugar, Arabic gum, mortar and pestle, water, cornstarch foil or wax paper.

Step 1: Gather all equipment and supplies that are required.

Step 2: Mix the desired medicated powder with confectioner's sugar (about 2 tablespoons of medicated powder per cup of confectioner's sugar) and several drops of gum Arabic powder in a mortar and pestle.

Step 3: Add a few drops of water at a time until you can form the mixture into a ball.

Step 4: Line a tray or plate with cornstarch and transfer the mixture to it.

Step 5: Flatten the ball to the desired thickness or make a long roll.

Step 6: Divide the mass into equal portions as desired.

Step 7: Allow the lozenges to air-dry or dry in a warm (not hot) oven.

Step 8: Wrap each lozenge in foil or wax paper after cooled.

COMPOUNDING OF SEMISOLID DRUGS

Ointments, creams, pastes, and gels may be intended for topical administration to skin or mucous membranes. Ointments are oil-based, while creams are water-based, but may be either oil-in-water or water-in-oil emulsions. Pastes contain a high proportion of solids, and gels are suspensions made of small inorganic or large organic particles mixed with a liquid. Generally, these dosage forms are applied externally. These types of agents include local antifungal agents, cortisol cream, and transdermal nitroglycerin.

Often, powdered or crystallized drugs are mixed into an ointment or a cream base in a mortar or on an ointment slab. These drugs include hydrocortisone, salicylic acid, and precipitated sulfur. Liquids may be incorporated by gradually adding them to an absorption-type base and then mixing thoroughly. Powders that are insoluble are first reduced to a fine powder and then added to the base (using the method of geometric dilution). Water-soluble substances may be dissolved with water and then added to the base. The final product of these types of compounded mixtures should be smooth, with no abrasive particles.

Ointments

An **ointment** is a highly viscous or semisolid substance used on the skin and may be referred to as an *emollient* or a *salve*. Ointments have an occlusive nature and hold water beneath the skin. They are most useful for the treatment of dermatologic conditions that include dry skin as part of the symptoms. Bases for ointments may be oil-in-water emulsions, water-in-oil emulsions, absorption bases, oleaginous bases, and water-soluble bases.

Procedure: Compounding an Ointment (or Cream)

Objective: To properly compound an ointment or cream.

Equipment Needed: balance, powder, mortar and pestle, compounding slab, ointment base, spatula, container, label.

Note: A cream is compounded in the same manner as the steps below, differing only in that the cream is water-based, while the ointment is oil-based.

Step 1: Gather all equipment and supplies that are required.

Step 2: Weigh the desired amount of powder to be mixed.

Step 3: Pour the powder into a mortar or onto a compounding slab to be mixed (Figure 5-7A).

Step 4: If the powder is not fine enough for mixing, triturate it until the particle sizes have been reduced.

Step 5: Add a partial amount of the ointment base and mix into the powder (Figure 5-7B).

Figure 5-7 Compounding an ointment. (A) Place powder onto ointment slab (B) Mix powder and cream.

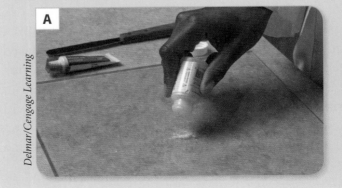
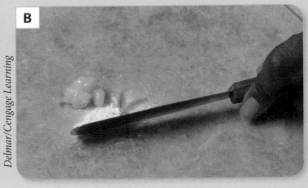

Delmar/Cengage Learning

Procedure: (Continued)

Figure 5-7 Compounding an ointment. (C) Ensure a smooth consistency (D) Place in container.

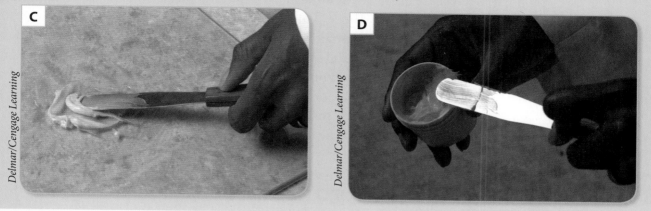

Delmar/Cengage Learning

Step 6: Continue adding the ointment base until the desired amount has been mixed with the powder.

Step 7: Confirm that the final mixture is very smooth, without any rough particles (Figure 5-7C).

Step 8: Transfer the mixture into the proper container (Figure 5-7D).

Step 9: Label the container properly. The ointment is now ready for dispensing to the patient.

Exercise: Compounding ointments

Objective: To be familiar with all equipment needed to compound ointments.

Gather all equipment required for compounding a jar of ointment.

Creams

Creams are pharmaceutical preparations that combine oil with water, and are usually used topically. They may or may not contain a medication. Creams are often dispensed in a tube or from a jar. They differ from lotions in that lotions contain more water, and are more fluid, while creams are thicker. The steps for compounding a cream are the same as those for compounding an ointment.

Pastes

A **paste** is a semisolid pharmaceutical preparation that is intended for external use. Some pastes contain a medication, while others are used for hygiene, such as toothpaste. Another example of this type of paste is 40% zinc oxide, which is used for diaper rash. Pastes do not melt or soften at body temperature. Pastes are similar to ointments, creams, and gels, differing in that they contain a higher proportion of solids. They are compounded in the same manner as ointments (above).

Gels

A **gel** is a jellylike substance commonly used for topical application that consists of particles mixed into a liquid, usually with an absorption base. Gels are classified as either inorganic two-phase systems or organic single-phase systems. Those that have large particle sizes in a two-phase system are known as **magmas**. Single-phase gels may have synthetic particles or may consist of natural mucilages or gums. The liquid portion may be water, alcohol, or of oleaginous origin. Most gels have absorption bases and are greaseless, water-absorbing, water-soluble, or water-washable. They are designed to have the same viscosity over many different temperatures. Gels are compounded in the same manner as ointments (above).

COMPOUNDING OF SUPPOSITORIES

Suppositories are available in various shapes, sizes, and weights. They may be used rectally or vaginally, or inserted into the urethra. Suppositories are used for both localized and systemic effects. The bases used for compounding suppositories are usually one of the following three substances: cocoa butter (theobroma oil), polyethylene glycol (Carbowax®), and glycerinated gelatin. Cocoa butter is usually used for rectal suppositories, while polyethylene glycol and glycerinated gelatin are suitable for both vaginal and rectal use.

To prepare suppositories, choose a proper mold, made of plastic, brass, rubber, stainless steel, or another suitable material. Suppositories are compounded by melting a base material, weighing a powdered medication, and adding the powder into the melted base. The two ingredients are then mixed together, and the mixture is poured into the suppository mold. Many suppository molds or containers are labeled "refrigerate" so that they retain their shape and effectiveness. No matter what type of base is used, suppositories should be kept in a cool, dry place prior to use.

Procedure: Compounding Suppositories

Objective: To properly compound suppositories.

Equipment Needed: balance, active ingredients, base material, beaker, heating device, spatula, suppository molds, container, label.

Step 1: Gather all equipment and supplies that are required.

Step 2: Weigh the desired amount of powder to be mixed into the suppository mixture.

Procedure: (Continued)

Step 3: Place the base material (which is commonly cocoa butter, a polyethylene glycol derivative, or glycerinated gelatin) into a beaker.

Step 4: Melt the base material over low heat (Figure 5-8A).

Step 5: Add the powder slowly into the melted base material (Figure 5-8B).

Step 6: Mix the two ingredients together, stirring until completely blended (Figure 5-8C).

Step 7: Pour the mixture into a suppository mold or molds (Figure 5-8D).

Step 8: Allow the suppositories to cool at room temperature for approximately 30 minutes.

Step 9: Place the suppositories in a refrigerator until they are cooled and relatively hardened.

Step 10: Place the completed suppositories in the proper container.

Step 11: Label the container correctly. The suppositories are now ready for dispensing to the patient.

Figure 5-8 Compounding suppositories. (A) Melt base material (B) Add powder to vase.

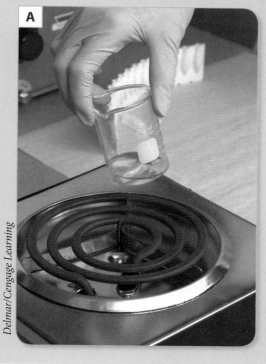

Delmar/Cengage Learning

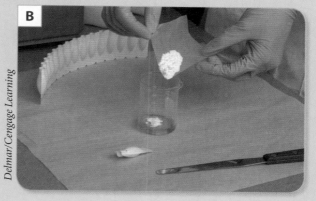

Delmar/Cengage Learning

Procedure: (Continued)

Figure 5-8 Compounding suppositories. (C) Stir (D) Add to suppository mold.

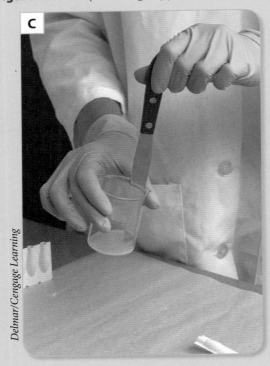

Delmar/Cengage Learning

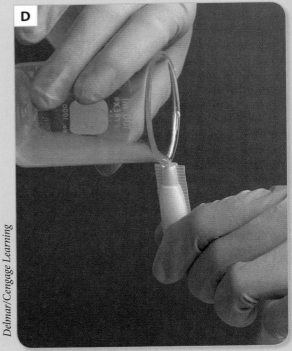

Delmar/Cengage Learning

COMPOUNDING OF LIQUID DRUGS

Liquid drugs are the most common form of compounded medications. To measure liquid drugs, familiarity with the following equipment is required:

- Conical graduates.
- Cylindrical graduates.
- Pipettes.

Solutions

A **solution** is a liquid dosage form containing active ingredients that are dissolved in a liquid vehicle, known as a **solvent**. The two types of solutions are as follows:

- Sterile parenteral and ophthalmic solutions.
- Nonsterile solutions (including oral, topical, and otic solutions).

Solutions are the simplest dosage forms compounded extemporaneously, as long as the following rules are followed:

- The solubility characteristics of each drug or chemical must be known so that each drug can be dissolved in the most soluble solvent.

- If an alcoholic solution of a drug that is poorly water-soluble is to be used, an aqueous solution will be added to maintain as high an alcohol concentration as possible.

- A drug's salt form (and not its free-acid or base form) is used because of higher solubility.

- When a salt is to be added to a syrup, the salt should first be dissolved in a few mL of water, and then the syrup should be added.

- The proper vehicle must be selected, whether it is an elixir, an aromatic or purified water, or a syrup.

- Flavoring or sweetening agents are prepared ahead of time.

Pharmacy technicians must not rush the compounding of solutions, taking the proper time to correctly complete the required procedure. They should gather all equipment ahead of time, including proper container sizes so that they will be at least half full when measuring solutions. A liquid's upper surface in a container is known as its *meniscus* (a moon-shaped body), wherein the liquid's upper edges will appear slightly higher than its center. Your eyes should be level with the liquid's top surface when measuring the liquid, with the level of the liquid at the bottom of the meniscus read to ensure an accurate measurement (Figure 5-9).

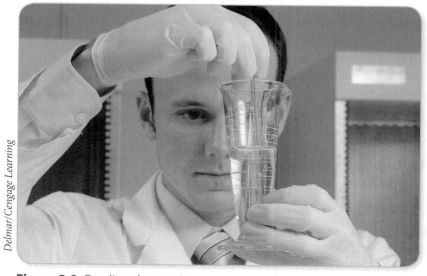

Delmar/Cengage Learning

Figure 5-9 Reading the meniscus.

Procedure: *Compounding Liquids*

Objective: To properly compound liquids.

Equipment Needed: active ingredients, graduate, container, label.

Step 1: Gather all equipment and supplies that are required.

Step 2: Slowly pour the liquid into the center of the graduate until you reach the desired volume.

Step 3: Allow enough time for the liquid to settle in the graduate before measuring.

Step 4: Measure the liquid by using the meniscus as discussed above.

Step 5: Pour the measured liquid into the desired container, completely draining all of it from the graduate.

Exercise: *The meniscus of a liquid*

Objective: To understand the importance of the meniscus of a liquid.

Measure 30mL, 50mL, and 75mL of any liquid by using its meniscus.

Suspensions

A **suspension** contains solid drug particles floating in a liquid medium which are easy to compound, but physically unstable. They must be shaken well before they are administered. When compounding a suspension, the insoluble powder(s) must be **triturated** (reduced to a fine powder by friction). Then, a small portion of liquid must be used to **levigate** the powder (grinding it in to a smooth surface with moisture). The powders are then triturated until a smooth paste is formed, with the levigating agent being added slowly as mixing continues. The vehicle containing the suspending agent is added in divided portions. A high-speed mixer may then be used to increase particle dispersion, with the completed suspension being labeled "Shake Well."

Procedure: *Compounding a Suspension*

Objective: To properly prepare a compounded suspension.

Equipment Needed: active ingredients, mortar and pestle, sieve, water or glycerin, graduate, spatula, container, label.

Step 1: Gather all equipment and supplies that are required.

Step 2: Grind the dry ingredients in a mortar with a pestle or use an electric grinder or blender (Figure 5-10A).

Step 3: Filter the pulverized powder through a 100-size mesh sieve.

Step 4: Wet the powder either with water (if it is hydrophilic and absorbs moisture easily) or with glycerin (if it is hydrophobic and repels water) (Figure 5-10B).

Step 5: Stir while continuing to add the correct wetting agent until it forms a thick paste.

Procedure: (Continued)

Step 6: Pour the mixture into a graduate.

Step 7: Add the remaining amount of wetting agent until the desired volume is reached.

Step 8: Stir the mixture until it is mixed evenly and thoroughly (use a homogenizer if needed to make particles as small as possible).

Step 9: Place the mixture in the appropriate container (Figure 5-10C).

Step 10: Label the container correctly, including a special label saying "Shake Well" (Figure 5-10D). The suspension is now ready for dispensing to the patient.

Figure 5-10 Compounding a suspension. (A) Crush ingredients (B) Add water (C) Pour mixture into bottle (D) Label.

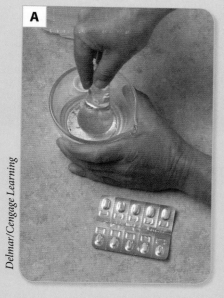

Delmar/Cengage Learning

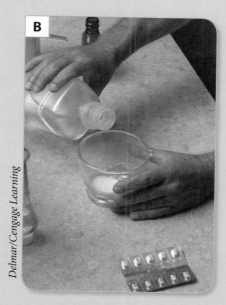

Delmar/Cengage Learning

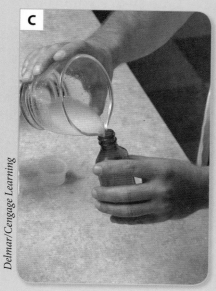

Delmar/Cengage Learning

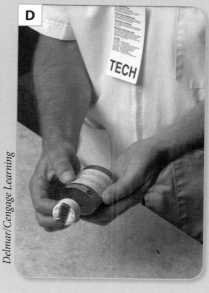

Delmar/Cengage Learning

Emulsions

An **emulsion** is a type of suspension that consists of two different liquids and an emulsifying agent (an *emulsifier*) that holds them together. There are two types, as follows:

- Oil-in-water (o/w) – usually for oral use, may be for external use; they are non-greasy, and easy to wash away using water—there is more water than oil in this type.

- Water-in-oil (w/o) – usually for external use; they are greasy and not easily washed away using water—there is more oil than water in this type.

There are two commonly used methods for making both types of emulsions: the "dry gum" (Continental) method and the wet gum" (English) method. The "dry gum" method is usually the preferred method.

Procedure: Dry Gum Method of Preparing an Emulsion

Objective: To properly compound an emulsion.

Equipment Needed: gum acacia, mortar and pestle, oil, water, active ingredients, graduate, container, label.

Step 1: Gather all equipment and supplies that are required.

Step 2: Pour the oil into the mortar (Figure 5-11A).

Step 3: Place the desired amount of gum acacia (also known as "gum Arabic") into the mortar (Figure 5-11B).

Figure 5-11 Compounding an emulsion – dry gum method. (A) Place oil into the mortar (B) Place gum into mortar.

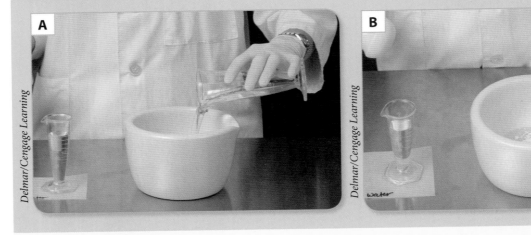

Delmar/Cengage Learning

Procedure: (Continued)

Step 4: Triturate the mixture until the acacia is thoroughly wet and smooth (Figure 5-11C).

Step 5: Measure the appropriate amount of water desired for the aqueous phase of the mixing in a clean graduate.

Step 6: Add all of the water at once (Figure 5-11D).

Step 7: Triturate the mixture with a hard and fast motion until the primary emulsion is formed; it will change from a translucent liquid to a white liquid, at which point the sound of the trituration will also change (Figure 5-11E).

Step 8: Add the other ingredients until the final desired volume is reached.

Step 9: Homogenize the preparation (Figure 5-11F).

Figure 5-11 Compounding an emulsion – dry gum method. (C) Triturate (D) Add water (E) Triturate (F) Homogenize.

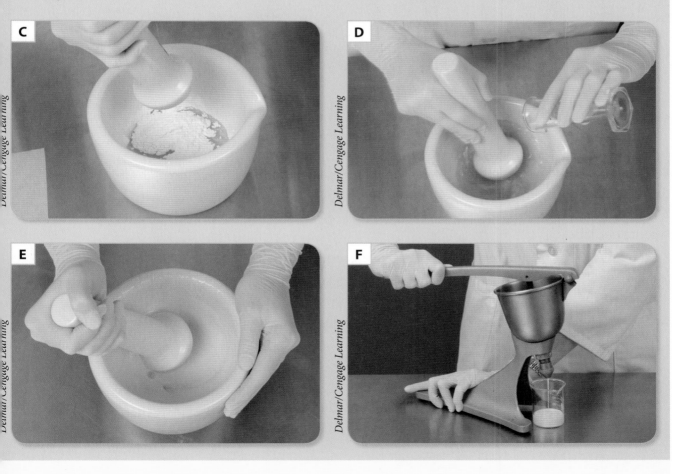

Procedure: (Continued)

Step 10: Place the mixture in the appropriate container (Figure 5-11G).

Step 11: Label the container correctly (Figure 5-11H). The emulsion is now ready to be dispensed to the patient.

Figure 5-11 Compounding an emulsion – dry gum method. (G) Place in appropriate container (H) Label the container.

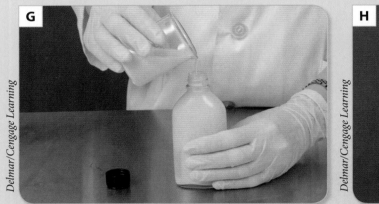
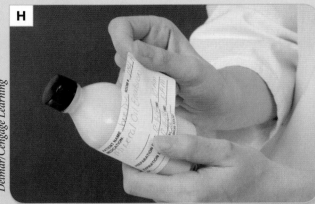

Procedure: *Wet Gum Method of Preparing an Emulsion*

Objective: To properly compound an emulsion.

Equipment Needed: gum acacia, mortar and pestle, glycerin, water, oil, active ingredients, graduate, container, label.

Step 1: Gather all equipment and supplies that are required.

Step 2: Place the desired amount of gum acacia (also known as "gum Arabic") into a Wedgwood mortar (Figure 5-12A).

Step 3: Gradually add in the desired amount of water while triturating the mixture (Figure 5-12B).

Figure 5-12 Compounding an emulsion – wet gum method. (A) Place gum into mortar (B) Add water and triturate.

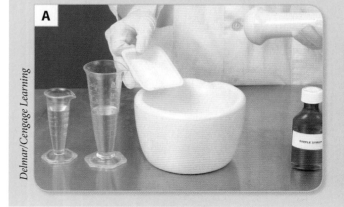
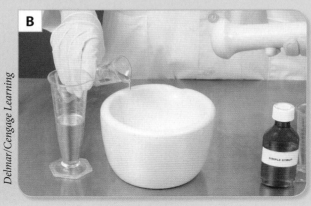

Procedure: (Continued)

Step 4: Gradually add in the desired amount of oil while triturating the mixture, until the primary mixture is formed (Figure 5-12C).

Step 5: Measure the syrup and active ingredient (Figure 5-12D).

Step 6: Add in any other ingredients (which may include water, water-soluble syrups, drugs, or chemicals) until the full desired volume is reached; in some cases, solid soluble ingredients must be dissolved in a suitable solvent before being added to the primary mixture (Figure 5-12E).

Step 7: Place the mixture in the appropriate container (Figure 5-12F).

Step 8: Label the container correctly (Figure 5-12G). The emulsion is now ready for dispensing to the patient.

Figure 5-12 Compounding an emulsion – wet gum method. (C) Add oil and triturate (D) Measure syrup and active ingredient (E) Add other ingredients (F) Place in appropriate container (G) Label the container.

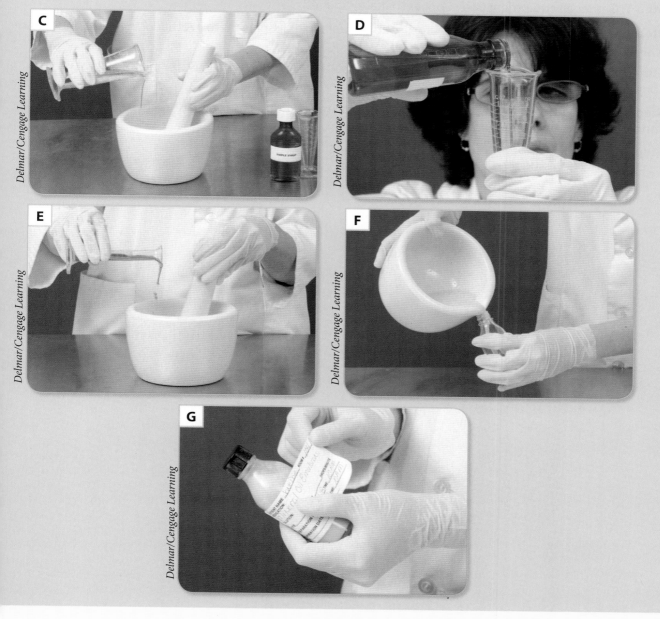

Delmar/Cengage Learning

Elixirs

Elixirs are liquid dosage forms that are sweetened and contain alcohol and water. These two liquid substances are known as a *co-solvent system.* Elixirs are made by dissolving alcohol-soluble ingredients in ethanol, and then dissolving water-soluble ingredients in water. Then, the two solvents are mixed together with constant stirring, adding the water (aqueous) component to the alcohol component.

Procedure: *Compounding an Elixir*

Objective: To properly compound an elixir.

Equipment Needed: active ingredients, ethanol, 2 glass containers, container, label.

Step 1: Gather all equipment and supplies that are required.

Step 2: Determine which ingredients are alcohol-soluble and dissolve them in ethanol in a glass container (Figure 5-13A).

Step 3: Determine which ingredients are water-soluble and dissolve them in water in a second glass container (Figure 5-13B).

Step 4: Add the water component into the alcohol mixture, stirring constantly (this keeps the alcohol concentration as strong as possible) (Figure 5-13C).

Step 5: Transfer to a proper container. Label the container.

Figure 5-13 Compounding an elixir. (A) Dissolve alcohol-soluble ingredients (B) Dissolve water-soluble ingredients (C) Add the two and triturate.

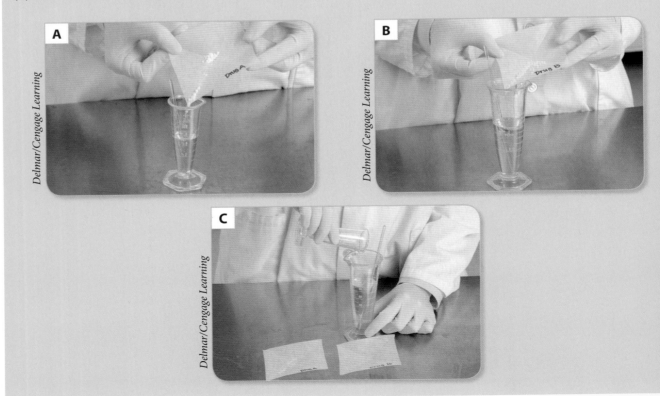

SUMMARY

Extemporaneous compounding helps to address the needs of patients that pre-manufactured pharmaceutical products do not meet. Technicians involved in pharmaceutical compounding must be fully trained and educated about this important task. Compounding may be done for solid drugs (tablets, capsules, and powders), semisolid drugs (ointments, creams, pastes, gels, and suppositories), and liquid drugs (solutions, suspensions, emulsions, and elixirs). Another type of solid drug is the lozenge (or troche). Liquid drugs are the most common form of compounded medications. Emulsions are commonly compounded using either the "wet gum" (English) method or the "dry gum" (Continental) method. The "dry gum" method is preferred.

REVIEW QUESTIONS

Multiple Choice

1. Which of the following dosage forms is contained in a gelatin shell?

   A. suppository   **C.** paste
   B. plaster   **D.** capsule

2. The smallest capsule is which of the following?

   A. 0   **C.** 3
   B. 1   **D.** 5

3. Which of the following may be a base for an ointment?

   A. oleaginous base   **C.** oil-in water emulsion
   B. water-in-oil emulsion **D.** all of the above

4. Suppositories containing cocoa butter are usually used for which of the following routes of administration?

   A. rectal   **C.** urethral
   B. vaginal   **D.** all of the above

5. Which of the following is the most common form of compounded medications?

   A. creams   **C.** liquid drugs
   B. capsules   **D.** tablets

6. Which of the following are the simplest dosage forms compounded extemporaneously?

   A. suspensions   **C.** emulsions
   B. solutions   **D.** elixirs

7. Which of the following dosage forms are made by compressing the powdered form of a drug with bulk filling material under high pressure?

    A. capsules
    B. pastes

    C. ointments
    D. tablets

8. Which of the following is an example of a soft-gelatin capsule?

    A. vitamin E
    B. mineral oil

    C. A and B
    D. none of the above

9. 40% zinc oxide, used for diaper rash, is an example of a:

    A. gel
    B. cream

    C. paste
    D. ointment

10. A liquid's upper surface in a container is called the:

    A. minim
    B. meniscus

    C. pastille
    D. paste

Fill in the Blank

1. Suppositories are compounded by melting a _____ material.

2. Gels are classified as either two-phase systems or organic _____ systems.

3. Creams differ from lotions in that lotions contain more _____.

4. When mixing heavier powders with lighter powders, the heavier powder should be placed _____ of the lighter powder and then blended.

5. Before capsules are filled with medication, the body and _____ of each capsule must be _____.

6. Capsule sizes range from number _____ (the smallest) to number _____ (the largest).

7. Special molds consisting of _____ and perforated _____ are used when manufacturing tablets.

8. Only properly educated and fully _____ pharmacy technicians should be involved in pharmaceutical compounding.

9. Caplets are tablets that are stamped into a _____ shape.

10. Long, thin, calibrated hollow glass tubes used for measurement of liquids less than 1.5 mL are called _____.

Repackaging and Labeling

OBJECTIVES

Upon completion of this chapter, the student should be able to:

1. Explain the factors required for special packaging.
2. List five advantages of repackaging bulk medications into unit-dose packages.
3. Demonstrate the proper handling of drugs during repackaging.
4. Define single-dose containers and single-unit containers.
5. Define heat-sealing systems and their classifications.
6. Describe labeling and record keeping.
7. Demonstrate record keeping and the use of repackaging logs and formulation records.
8. Demonstrate the appropriate storage of medications by checking their labels.

GLOSSARY

Blister package – A type of medication packaging that features a hollow plastic/PVC portion containing the medication, which is backed by a paper or foil backing that peels off from the "blister" portion.

Pouch package – A type of medication packaging that consists of clear or light-resistant plastic/PVC bags which are sealed with an adhesive.

Repackaging – The breaking down of bulk medications into smaller packages for specific use, such as unit-dose packages.

Tyvek® – A type of material used in certain medication packages; it consists of a very strong and impervious spun polythene material.

Unit-dose – Systems that contain medication in a single-unit package intended for single-dose administration to a patient.

Vaginal syringes – Applicators used to instill vaginal creams and gels directly into the vagina; they consist of applicators with plungers intended for one-time use.

OVERVIEW

Repackaging and labeling are sometimes necessary when required dosage forms are not available commercially. The pharmacy technician may be directly involved in preparing unit-dose packaging using automated packaging equipment. The pharmacy technician must be adequately trained to ensure the stability of the product and appropriate labeling.

Depending on the product, the method of dispensing, and the desired route of administration, there are different container types from which to choose, which include unit-dose packaging for solid oral forms (tray-filled blister packaging) and oral liquids (oral syringes). In addition, some of the new automated dispensing technologies require packaging unique to their dispensing design.

REPACKAGING OF DRUGS

Alert

- It is important to inform the pharmacy technician in training that the industry has been adjusting to "unit of use" labels for oral, injectable, and external products.

- Where repacks are used, the labels are cumbersome (but mandated by state and federal regulations).

- When repackaged pharmaceuticals expire, they cannot be returned and must be disposed of.

Repackaging is the breaking down of bulk medications into smaller packages for specific use, such as unit-dose packages. Repackaging records are used when repackaging drugs in a pharmacy. These records include the name, lot number, quantity, strength, manufacturer's name, distributor's name, repacking date, number of packages prepared, number of dosage units in each package, signature of the person performing the repackaging, signature of the supervising pharmacist, and any other required identifying marks. Repackaging records are used when a drug recall occurs to determine if the recalled drug has been repackaged. Federal law requires that the expiration dates of repackaged drugs be 6 months or less. This period cannot be more than 25 percent of the time remaining according to the original bulk container expiration date. An example of a repackaging record is shown in Figure 6-1.

Exercise

Objective: To understand the needs required for keeping records of repackaged drugs.

Select 10 different repackaged drugs and write down all the information that is required for a repackaging record.

FLORIDA MEDICAL CENTER

REPACKAGING RECORD

MPI UNIT-DOSE SYSTEM

PACKAGING DATES FROM: 08/11/2008 to 99/99/9999

	TITLE / MANUFACTURER		BEYOND-USE M-EXPIRY#	LOT M-LOT	QUAN
1	BUPROPION S.R. 150 MG S.R. TAB		08/11/2009	3889	
	08/11/2008 TEVA	ALA BCD	09/30/2009	7092161	100
2	DILTIAZEM CD 240 MG CAP		08/11/2009	3890	
	08/11/2008 ACTAVIS LLC	ALA BCD	11/30/2009	710C81	30
3	GUAIFENESIN L.A. 600 MG S.R. TAB		08/11/2009	3886	
	08/11/2008 ADAMS	ALA BCD	02/28/2011	PL00007301	40
4	PRAVASTATIN 20 MG TAB		08/11/2009	3887	
	08/11/2008 TEVA	ALA BCD	06/30/2010	P29152	100
5	TOPIRAMATE 25 MG TAB		08/11/2009	3888	
	08/11/2008 ORTHO MCNEIL	ALA BCD	03/31/2010	8EG527	60
6	ZONISAMIDE 25 MG CAP		01/31/2009	3885	
	08/11/2008 APOTEX	ALA BCD	01/31/2009	HG5815	100

—REPORT SUMMARY—

TIMES PACKED = 6
UNITS PACKED = 430

FIRST JOB = 08/11/2008
LAST JOB = 08/11/2008

Figure 6-1 A sample repackaging record.

SPECIAL PACKAGING REQUIREMENTS

Certain drugs have special packaging requirements according to the United States Pharmacopoeia (USP) and National Formulary (NF), including:

- Hermetic containers, which are impervious to air or any other gas during handling, shipment, storage, and distribution.

- Light-resistant containers, which use special materials and coatings that are usually opaque to protect from light that may damage the substances contained within; usually, special labeling is added that reads "protect from light."

- Single-dose containers, used for parenteral products only; these include pre-filled syringes, cartridges, closure-sealed containers, and fusion-sealed containers.

- Single-unit containers, which hold drug products intended for administration as a single dose, or a single finished device that must be used immediately after the container is opened; these containers must be labeled to indicate the contained substance's identity, quantity, manufacturer name, lot number, expiration date, and strength.

- Tamper-resistant packaging, used for sterile ophthalmic or otic products, or for items requiring immediate extemporaneous compounding; they are sealed so that they cannot be opened without visible destruction of the container's seal.

- Tight containers, which can be tightly re-closed and protect from contamination, spillage, and evaporation.

- Unit-dose containers, which are single-unit containers used for non-parenteral articles intended for administration direct from the container.

UNIT-DOSE SYSTEM

Unit-dose systems contain medication in a single-unit package intended for single-dose administration to a patient. They are dispensed from a pharmacy requiring no further preparation before use by the patient. Unit-dose packaging consists of many forms such as plastic packs, tubes, ampules, and vials (Figure 6-2). Pharmacy technicians spend much of their time working with unit-dose systems. Advantages of the unit-dose system include reduction of medication errors, decrease in costs, better patient care, better monitoring of drug use, more accurate billing, reduction of drug credits, lowered inventories, and reduction of wasted drugs. Unit doses are

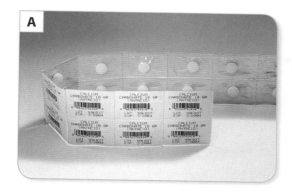

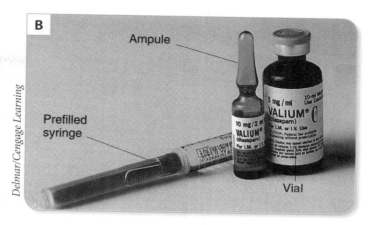

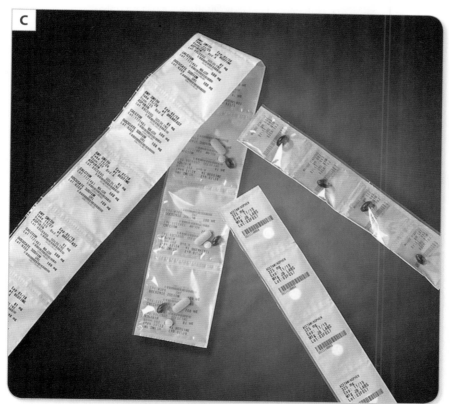

Figure 6-2 (A) Unit-dose package (B) Pre-filled syringe and single-dose ampule and vial (C) Multiple-medication package. (Courtesy of AutoMed Technologies, Inc.)

Alert

Some medications, including creams, eye drops, and metered-dose inhalers, cannot be divided into unit doses.

taken to nursing stations in individual drawers or trays in a medication cart—one drawer for each patient's daily medication needs (Figures 6-3 and 6-4). Pharmacy technicians may manually fill these cart drawers or use machinery for the same task. Each drawer is labeled with a specific patient's name and room number. The supervising pharmacist must check the accuracy of the filling of each drawer with the proper medications. Drawers for unit doses may be updated as needed during each day.

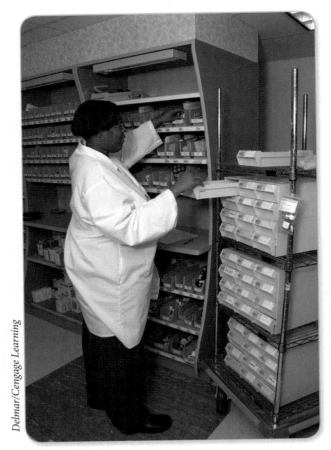

Delmar/Cengage Learning

Figure 6-3 Medication carts.

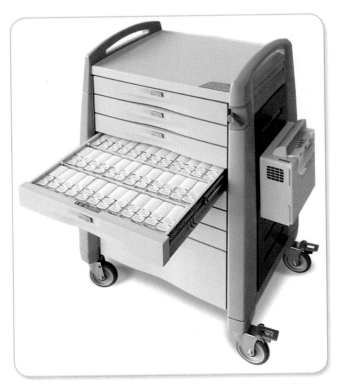

Figure 6-4 Medication cart. (Courtesy of Artromick International, Inc.)

Exercise

Objective: To become familiar with the filling of a medication cart.

Choose an empty tray from a medication cart and fill it with 10 unit doses of medication. Label the empty tray with a fictional patient's name.

Single-Unit Packaging

Single-unit packaging consists of a single dosage form. This includes one tablet, one capsule, or one tablespoon of a liquid medication. Both single-unit and single-dose packages (which are defined below) have reduced the need for pharmacy technicians to repackage medications from manufacturers.

Single-Dose Packaging

Single-dose packaging is not the same as single-unit packaging. If two tablets are required for a "single dose" of medication, then a single-dose package would contain these two tablets (see Figure 6-2B). "Single-dose" is defined as the amount of medication, regardless of count, that is required for a single dose for a patient. Most but not all medications are available in single-dose packaging, requiring the repackaging of some medications by pharmacy technicians into single-dose containers.

REPACKAGING EQUIPMENT

Equipment for repackaging includes different containers, including medication vials, bags, bottles, heat-sealed containers, syringes, and ampules. Repackaging equipment can be fully automated, semi-automated, or manual. The more manual the system used, the greater the chance of the packaging being compromised, increasing the chance for contamination or alteration of the drug product. Since most doses dispensed in institutions are oral solids, more repackaging systems are available for these medications than for any other dosage form.

PACKAGING OF ORAL SOLID SYSTEMS

The two types of oral solid packaging are **blister packages** and **pouch packages**. Containers for packaging may be made of plastic or glass. Prior to the recognition of the use of plastics in health care practice, glass was the predominant material used in the primary packaging of pharmaceutical products. Glass has several advantages, which include:

- It is relatively unreactive and an inert substance.

- It can be used in contact with many critical products, either dry or liquid.

- It provides excellent protection against water vapor and gas permeation.

- It can withstand steam sterilization (autoclaving) without incurring physical distortion.

Disadvantages of glass in the field of packaging include its fragility and weight.

Blister system packages (plastic blisters or bubble packages) are usually made of polyvinyl chloride (PVC) plastic. They may be composed of paper or foil backing that peels off from the blister portion of the packaging. The blister tray is subsequently sealed to a **Tyvek**® or paper lid. Either type of lid material is a sterile barrier and permits steam to penetrate the package. Blister packages are more rigid than pouch packages, and are used with some manually operated repackaging systems.

Pouch systems consist of clear or light-resistant plastic/PVC bags. Oral solids are dropped into the bag, which is sealed with an adhesive. Pouch systems are easily repackaged using automated machinery. Figure 6-5 shows an example of a punch card.

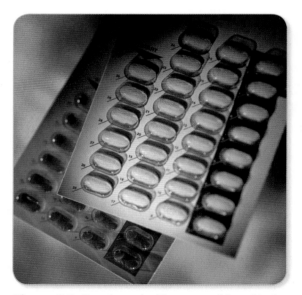

Figure 6-5 Punch cards. (Courtesy of AutoMed Technologies, Inc.)

Manually operated oral solid repackaging systems are used for both blister and pouch packaging. They may use either heat or adhesive sealing methods. Heat-sealing systems produce Class A through D packages, while adhesive sealing systems produce B through D packages.

Automated oral solid repackaging systems produce pouch packages by feeding oral solids into a wheel that drops the dose into the pouch. Two heated wheels then seal each pouch. Automated repackaging machinery can package up to 120 doses of a single drug per minute. Penicillins and oncolytic drugs should not be packaged in automated systems in order to avoid contamination of the equipment (Figure 6-6).

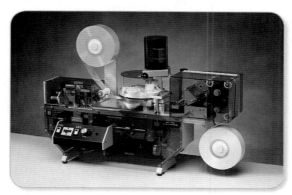

Figure 6-6 Unit-dose packaging machine. (Courtesy of AutoMed Technologies, Inc.)

PACKAGING OF ORAL LIQUID SYSTEMS

Oral liquid repackaging uses both manual and automated systems. Manual systems use glass or plastic vials or syringes, while automated systems use plastics exclusively.

Manual repackaging systems for oral liquids use glass or plastic vials, or glass or plastic syringes. Closure systems include screw caps, permanently affixed tops, and crimped caps. Liquids may be transferred into a beaker and withdrawn into a syringe for repackaging, or spring-loaded syringes may be used. Another manual method of repackaging oral liquids involves the use of burettes instead of syringes. In this method, a specially designed cap on the bulk liquid bottle allows a syringe to be inserted and the liquid withdrawn.

Automated liquid repackaging systems use plastic cups as fluid reservoirs and PVC/paper/foil seals. Peristaltic pumps deliver the correct amount of fluid into each cup. The overseal is attached by using heat and pressure. These machines can produce up to 32 units per minute, in sizes that range from 15 to 45 mL. These machines produce packages with a Class A rating.

Alert

The supervising pharmacist must verify the accuracy of functions involving repackaging and labeling as conducted by the pharmacy technician.

COMMONLY REPACKAGED DRUGS

Oral liquids and topical medications are commonly repackaged products, usually using glass or plastic containers, which are explained in detail below.

Oral Liquids

Oral liquids are commonly repackaged in glass or plastic oral vials or syringes. Plastics have become more prevalent as they have become improved, cheaper, lighter than glass, and durable. Glass or plastic vials are still most frequently used to contain oral liquids. They usually feature rubber stopper or metal screw caps. Plastic vials are often fitted with plastic balls that fit int small filling holes located at the bottom of the vials. Oral syringes are simila to injectable syringes, and are composed of either glass or plastic.

Topical Drugs

Topical drugs (usually ointments or creams) are commonly repackage into glass or plastic tubes or jars. Vaginal creams and gels are ofte repackaged into **vaginal syringes**, usually with tube adapters that allow an size tube that may be required.

LABELING

Labels contain information and instructions, and are attached t medication containers to identify the contents inside. For example, the lab for a bottle of regular-strength aspirin would identify the contents as aspirin 325 mg (Figure 6-7).

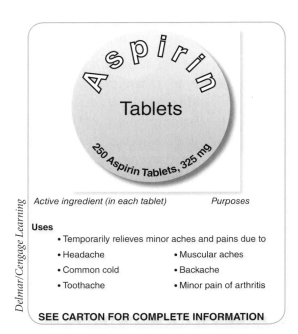

Delmar/Cengage Learning

Figure 6-7 Aspirin label.

Correct labeling should be verified by the person handling th dispensing of drugs. Computers now play a large part in assuring tha correct labeling and packaging of drug products occurs. Medication label must be computer-generated, machine-printed, or typed. Control or lo numbers should always appear on package labeling. Labeling guns may b used to semi-automate the process of labeling drug containers. Pharmac technicians are often responsible for labeling medications. The supervisin pharmacist must confirm that the labeling has been done correctly.

Standard medication labels should include the pharmacy's or other institution's name, address, and phone number. Accessory labeling must be used when special instructions are indicated, such as "Keep Refrigerated" or "Shake Well." Every therapeutically active ingredient must be listed on the label. Expiration dates must be included.

Alert

Verify all components of each drug label to make sure that they exactly match the prescription order. Handwritten labels are prohibited and writing by hand on a medication label must be avoided.

Exercise

Objective: To become familiar with the information that is needed to document records in the computer system and to create labels.

Choose 5 packages of oral solids and 5 packages of oral liquid medications, and enter all of the information from these packages into a computer system. Then, print the labels in the pharmacy laboratory.

RECORD KEEPING

The maintenance of accurate and complete records of the entire repackaging process is essential for correct management of inventory and for achieving efficiency. Pharmacy technicians play a large part in correct record-keeping practices during repackaging. Most record keeping is now done on computers, including daily repackaging logs, formulation records, and prepackaging records. Formulation records include labeling information, the type of container used, processing equipment used, drug stability information, and lists of any hazardous materials involved in the process. Repackaging records include the drug's name, strength, dosage form, date of repackaging, manufacturer's information, lot number, beyond-use date, and repackaging information.

Exercise

Objective: To become familiar with the information needed for a repackaging record.

Write the information from 5 medication containers into a repackaging record.

STORAGE

After drugs have been repackaged, they must be properly stored. Appropriate storage requires environmental, security, and safety considerations. Certain medications require storage that includes freezing, refrigeration, light-protection, or room-temperature conditions. Manufacturer's requirements must be followed so that the medication's safety and effectiveness are not compromised. In the hospital pharmacy, when unused stock is returned from nursing stations, it should be put back into place as soon as possible by pharmacy technicians. Certain toxic chemicals should be kept inside cabinets and kept low to the ground; they should never be stored out in the open. The proper storage of every substance in the pharmacy is the responsibility of all pharmacy employees.

Exercise

Objective: To become familiar with the storage requirements of various pharmaceuticals and how to obtain that information.

Read the labels of 6 medications and demonstrate how to properly store them.

SUMMARY

Repackaging and labeling is required for some dosage forms that are not available commercially. Pharmacy technicians must be trained in these tasks and be familiar with different methods of repackaging and labeling as well as with the variety of equipment and containers that is required. Certain drugs have special packaging requirements such as hermetic containers, light-resistant containers, single-dose containers, tamper-resistant packaging, and "tight" containers.

Unit-dose systems contain medication in a single-unit package intended for single-dose administration to a patient. Repackaging for oral solid or oral liquid systems may be conducted manually or by using automated equipment. Oral liquids and topical medications are commonly repackaged products, which usually use glass or plastic containers.

Labeling of containers is essential for accurate repackaging, and must contain all drug information as well as lot numbers. Another important factor in the process of repackaging is record keeping, which must be accurate and complete.

REVIEW QUESTIONS

Multiple Choice

1. Automated systems for oral liquid repackaging use which of the following containers exclusively?

   A. plastic
   B. glass

   C. either plastic or glass
   D. neither plastic or glass

2. Automated liquid repackaging machines can produce up to how many units per minute?

   A. 12
   B. 32

   C. 48
   D. 100

3. Which of the following should always appear on the package labeling?

   A. name of manufacturer
   B. name of pharmacist
   C. license number
   D. lot number

4. Repackaging records include all of the following information, except:

   A. license number of the pharmacy technician
   B. lot number
   C. date of repackaging
   D. signature of the supervising pharmacist

5. Which of the following types of containers are used for oral liquids?

    A. tray-filled blister packages
    B. unit-dose packages
    C. oral syringes
    D. all of the above

6. Tamper-resistant packaging is used for which of the following medications?

    A. capsules and tablets
    B. syrups
    C. sterile ophthalmics
    D. all of the above

7. All of the following are advantages of the unit-dose system, except:

    A. decrease in costs
    B. increase in costs
    C. reduction of medication errors
    D. better patient care

8. The blister tray is subsequently sealed to which of the following?

    A. paper lid   C. Tyvek lid
    B. pouches   D. A and C

9. Light-resistant PVC bags are called:

    A. oral liquid systems
    B. pouch systems
    C. blister package systems
    D. none of the above

10. Appropriate storage requires which of the following?

    A. security measures
    B. environmental temperature control
    C. safety measures
    D. all of the above

Fill in the Blank

1. Most record keeping is now done on _____.

2. Lot numbers should always appear on package _____.

3. Vaginal creams are often repackaged into _____ syringes.

4. Automated repackaging machinery can package up to _____ doses of a single drug per minute.

5. Heat-sealing systems produce Class A through Class _____ packages.

6. Disadvantages of glass in packaging include its fragility and _____.

7. Single-dose packaging is not the same as single-_____ packaging.

8. Single-unit packaging consists of a _____ form.

9. Tight containers protect from contamination, _____, and _____.

10. When repackaged pharmaceuticals expire, they must be _____ of.

STERILE COMPOUNDING PRODUCTS

Aseptic Techniques and Clean Rooms

OBJECTIVES

Upon completion of this chapter, the student should be able to:

1. Identify bacteria and viruses, as well as describe some of their characteristics.
2. Outline the methods of transmission of infection.
3. Explain the ways in which infectious diseases are spread.
4. Describe the principles of asepsis.
5. Explain the importance of hand washing in control of infectious diseases.
6. Describe the clean room in the pharmacy setting and its purpose.
7. Explain laminar-airflow hoods.
8. Identify vertical and horizontal laminar-airflow hoods.

GLOSSARY

Asepsis – The process of inhibiting the growth and multiplication of microorganisms.

Autoclave – High-heat, high-pressure device used to sterilize equipment.

Bacteria – Simple one-celled microbes that are named according to their shapes and arrangement; they cause infections throughout the body.

Cleaning – Physical removal of soil, blood, and debris from instruments and other items.

Clean technique – Use of practices such as hand washing, general cleaning, and disinfection to reduce the presence of pathogenic microorganisms; also known as *medical asepsis.*

Disinfection – Destruction of pathogenic microorganisms by exposure to chemicals or physical agents.

Flora – Microbial organisms occurring naturally in the body.

Infection – The invasion of the body by pathogenic microorganisms and their multiplication, which can lead to tissue damage and disease.

Medical asepsis – Use of practices such as hand washing, general cleaning, and disinfection to reduce the presence of pathogenic microorganisms; also known as *clean technique.*

Microbes – Minute life forms; especially disease-causing bacteria.

Microbiology – The branch of biology that studies microorganisms and their effects on humans.

Microorganisms – Minute life forms that are invisible to the naked eye; they include both free-living and parasitic life forms.

Nosocomial infection – Infection acquired in a hospital or institutional environment

Sodium hypochlorite – The least expensive and most readily available chemical for cleaning surfaces; it is also known as *ordinary household bleach.*

Transmission – A passage or transfer, as of a disease from one individual to another.

Virus – A microorganism smaller than a bacterium, which cannot grow or reproduce apart from a living cell.

OVERVIEW

It is essential to ensure that proper aseptic technique be used for the preparation of safe and effective sterile pharmaceutical compounding. Aseptic technology is the application of scientific understanding of the characteristics of viable microorganisms, applied in such a manner that the microorganisms are eliminated, with a high probability of success, from all of the process steps involved in compounding sterile pharmaceutical dosage forms.

Regardless of where aseptic processing (compounding) is practiced—in an institutional setting, a home infusion pharmacy, or a pharmaceutical manufacturing facility—the principles are the same; only the practices differ. Practices will differ because of the nature of the product being produced, the size of the batch, the length of the projected shelf life, and the extent of the regulatory requirements involved.

Pharmacy technicians who are trained to deal with pharmaceutical compounding must understand basic **microbiology**, methods of disease **transmission**, and principles of asepsis. They must also be familiar with clean rooms and clean air environments. The technician needs to understand the goal of laminar-airflow hoods and follow the policy and regulation of working in clean rooms to reduce the risk of bacterial contamination.

MICROORGANISMS

Microorganisms, minute life forms that are invisible to the naked eye, are a natural part of the world in which we live. There are many different types of microorganisms, including bacteria, viruses, fungi, and protozoa. The microorganisms that are most important to guard against in the clean room when dealing with aseptic techniques are bacteria and viruses.

Bacteria

Bacteria are one-celled **microbes** that are named according to shape and arrangement. Many bacteria reside naturally within the human body and cause no disease unless the opportunity arises. Therefore, they are referred

to as "opportunistic" microbes. For example, *E. coli* resides in the lumen o
the intestine in humans. This bacterium is capable of causing infection whe
released into the peritoneal cavity. Some bacteria are pathogens and ma
cause infections throughout the body, including the respiratory tract, skin
bloodstream, and urinary tract. Each genus of bacteria has a characteristi
shape that can aid in identification: round, rod, or spiral (Figure 7-1)

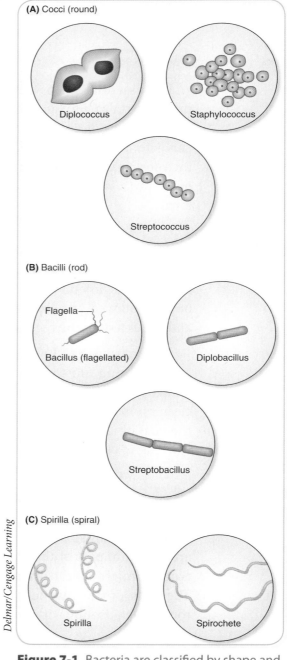

Figure 7-1 Bacteria are classified by shape and
arrangement: round, rod, or spiral in shape, and
arranged as clusters (staphylococcus), chains
(streptococcus), or paired (diplobacillus).

Bacteria grow in *colonies,* which are groups that are usually arranged as follows:

- Chains (streptococci).

- Clusters (staphylococci).

- Pairs (diplococci).

Exercise

Objective: To familiarize oneself with the various forms of bacteria.

Identify different bacterial microorganisms according to their shape and arrangement by using pre-prepared microscope slides.

Viruses

Unlike bacteria, which are living microorganisms, viruses are non-living particles that are completely reliant on a host cell for survival. A **virus** is the smallest type of microbe. Viruses exist in numerous shapes and are classified according to the following characteristics:

- Clinical properties.

- Type of nucleic acid core (either deoxyribonucleic acid (DNA) and ribonucleic acid (RNA).

Common viral infections include the following:

- Hepatitis.

- Herpes.

- Chickenpox.

- Human immunodeficiency virus (HIV).

- Common cold.

- Influenza.

- Measles.

- Mumps.

The chances of contamination with other microorganisms, such as parasites or fungi, are very rare. Therefore, discussion of them is not necessary in this text.

Types of Infections

Infections may be:

- Generalized – such as pneumonia in the lungs.
- Local – such as boils or skin abscesses; confined to one area of the body.
- Systemic – widespread throughout the bloodstream; known as *bacteremia.*

Normal body **flora** (microbial organisms occurring naturally within the body) lives in and on our body surfaces, differing in each area of the body. Normal body flora may become unbalanced because of:

- Entrance of pathogenic organisms.
- Moving to a new area of the body where they don't normally exist.
- Use of antibiotics, which can upset normal balances of flora; this allows one group of flora to grow and flourish.

Methods of Transmission

Any **infection** (tissue damage or disease related to pathogenic microorganisms) requires a primary agent, such as a bacterium, virus, fungus, or parasite. Frequent hand washing helps to eliminate transient microbes from the skin, thereby reducing the risk of infection. In the pharmacy, compounding of different substances (which may be sterile or nonsterile) can become contaminated with pathogenic microorganisms and cause infection.

The following are facts that pharmacy technicians must remember:

- The primary mode of airborne bacteria in pharmacy compounding is from the individuals who are dealing with the compounding of medications.
- Pharmacy technicians may disperse microorganisms from their own skin.
- Most problems occur because of contamination during the procedure.

The sources of contamination can be divided into two groups: environmental and endogenous. Environmental sources include personnel, the environment, and contaminated instrumentation. Endogenous sources come from agents within the host itself.

Personnel

Pharmacy technicians will focus on their hands during sterile compounding, and a large part of compounding awareness concerns proper hand hygiene and the proper wearing of intact gloves to prevent skin contamination. The skin and hair of pharmacy technicians are reservoirs of bacteria, which may be shed in particle form into the air, and therefore pose a risk of sterile compounding site infection to the patient. Personnel are required to wear gowns, gloves, caps, and masks when dealing with sterile compounding. This is discussed further in Chapter 8.

Environment

A second source of microbial transmission is environmental, from both fomites (pathogens on inanimate objects) and through the air. A safe and spacious clean room helps to provide a lower level of microbes in the environment. For example, a clean room is designed with a clean zone, filtered and controlled air systems, and soil-resistant building materials. This type of clean room design has become routine in sterile compounding. The clean room requires personnel to follow strict cleanliness procedures, which are very effective in preventing contamination.

Within the clean room environment, the patient is at risk of infection from airborne pathogens. The clean room is designed to minimize this via the use of laminar-airflow systems (which are discussed later in this chapter). Fomites can exist on walls, floors, cabinets, furniture, and nonsterile supplies.

Instruments

Contamination of instruments may also result from the improper cleaning or decontamination of compounding equipment, IV lines, and fluids. The use of nonsterile medications poses a risk of infection to the patient.

PRINCIPLES OF ASEPSIS

The safety of the patient depends on strict adherence by pharmacy technicians to sterile technique. Technicians must also be constantly aware of the sterile technique of other personnel within the clean room. Adherence to the principles of **asepsis** reflects the pharmacy technician's compounding conscience and ability to assist in preventing contaminations. This will result in a lower risk of harm to patients.

MEDICAL ASEPSIS

Asepsis is the absence of disease-producing microorganisms, which can be achieved by medical aseptic technique and surgical aseptic technique. **Medical asepsis** is the use of practices such as hand washing, general cleaning, and disinfecting contaminated surfaces while adhering to Standard and Transmission-Based Precautions. These measures are aimed at destroying pathologic organisms after they leave the body. These techniques are used to decrease the risk for transmission of contaminants to others. Medical aseptic technique is sometimes called **clean technique**. Articles that have contacted known pathogens or have been exposed to potential pathogens are referred to as *contaminated* or *dirty*, while articles that are free of pathogens are referred to as *uncontaminated* or *clean*.

Microbes may be reduced by using medical aseptic technique, which includes:

- Regular hand washing.
- Using nonsterile gloves (especially when in contact with blood, body fluids, mucous membranes, or non-intact skin).
- Proper cleaning and disinfecting of equipment.

A list of commonly used antiseptics, disinfectants, and sterilizing agents, and their areas of application, is shown in Table 7-1.

TABLE 7-1 Antiseptics, Disinfectants, and Sterilizing Agents

Compound	Common Usage
Antiseptics	
Glycerol (50%)	Stool and surgical specimens
Hydrogen peroxide (3%)	Skin infections
Iodine (tincture in alcohol)	Skin
Iodophors	Skin
Isopropyl alcohol (70%)	Skin
Potassium permanganate	Urethral, skin fungus infections
Silver nitrate (1%)	Eye infections in newborns
Zinc oxide paste	Diaper rash
Zinc salts of fatty acids	Athlete's foot
Disinfectants	
Formaldehyde (4%)	Thermometers
Hexachlorophene	Pre-surgical hand washing
Iodine (1% in 70% alcohol)	External surfaces
Iodophors	External surfaces and thermometers
Lysol (5%)	External surfaces
Phenol (5%)v	External surfaces
Sodium hypochlorite (5%)	External surfaces
Zephrin (0.001%)	Thermometers

TABLE 7-1   Antiseptics, Disinfectants, and Sterilizing Agents (*continued*)

Compound	Common Usage
Sterilizing Agents	
Ethylene oxide gas (12%)	Linens and equipment
Formaldehyde (20% in 70% alcohol)	Metal instruments
Glutaraldehyde (more than 7.5 pH)	Metal instruments

Hand Hygiene

Hand hygiene is the most important health procedure that can be performed to prevent the spread of microbes of all types. It requires washing the hands by vigorous rubbing of all surfaces of the hands while lathered with an appropriate antimicrobial soap (from a dispenser, and not in bar form), followed by rinsing under running, warm water. Cold water does not provide enough lather from the soap and hot water may damage the skin.

Since faucets may be a source for contamination, a paper towel should be used to turn faucets on and off, or a knee or foot pedal should be used to control the flow of water. While washing, always keep the fingertips pointed downward, never lean against the sink, and never touch the inside of the sink. The friction created by rubbing the hands together during washing mechanically removes microbes from the hands, and along with proper soap and running water, is the most significant way to prevent **nosocomial infections** (those that can be acquired by caring for patients in health care facilities). Likewise, proper hand hygiene is the single most important control measure to break the chain of infection.

Procedure: Hand Washing

Objective: To use proper technique during hand hygiene procedures to reduce the spread of infection.

Equipment Needed: sink, running water, antimicrobial liquid soap, a nail brush (or orange stick), paper towels within a dispenser, water-based antimicrobial lotion, and a properly labeled biohazard waste container.

Step 1: Remove all jewelry.

Step 2: Turn on the water faucets with a paper towel if they are not foot-operated.

Step 3: Make sure that the water is lukewarm.

Step 4: Wet your hands.

Step 5: Apply soap and lather with a circular motion and friction, holding the fingertips downward (Figure 7-2A).

Step 6: Make sure to rub well between the fingers.

Procedure: *(Continued)*

Step 7: If this is the first time of the day you are washing your hands, use a nail brush (or orange stick) to clean under every fingernail.

Step 8: Rinse well while holding the hands with the fingertips still pointed downward (Figure 7-2B).

Step 9: Repeat the scrubbing procedure a second time, for 1 to 2 minutes.

Step 10: Rinse again.

Step 11: Dry hands with paper towels, avoiding touching the paper towel dispenser (Figure 7-2C).

Step 12: Turn off the water faucets with a paper towel if they are not foot-operated (Figure 7-2D).

Step 13: Place used towels in the biohazard waste container.

Step 14: Apply the water-based antibacterial hand lotion to prevent chapping or drying of the skin.

Figure 7-2 Hand washing technique. (A) Lather hands with soap and firmly rub all surfaces (B) Rinse hands with fingers pointing down (C) Dry hands with paper towel (D) Turn water off with paper towel.

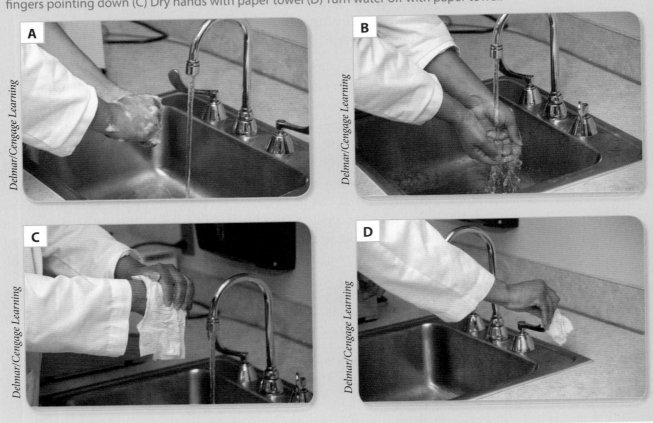

Exercise : Hand hygiene

Objective: To reinforce the importance of hand hygiene.

Practice the procedure of hand washing.

The hands can usually be washed effectively in 15 to 20 seconds unless they are visibly dirty or soiled. The hands must be washed at all of the following times:

- When beginning a shift.

- Before handling any food or drinks.

- After picking up anything from the floor.

- After using the bathroom.

- After coughing, sneezing, or using a tissue for any reason.

- After handling any items belonging to a patient.

- After touching any surfaces that patients may have touched or that may be soiled for any reason.

- Before handling any item or supply that is considered clean.

- Immediately before touching the mucous membranes or non-intact skin.

- Immediately after contact with blood, moist body fluids, mucous membranes, or non-intact skin.

- Before and after any contact with your own mouth or mucous membranes.

- Before and after any contact with any patient.

- Before applying and after removing gloves.

- Whenever the hands are visibly dirty.

- Any time gloves get torn.

- When finishing a shift.

For further hygiene, it is recommended that the nails are kept short and artificial nails are not worn. Real or artificial nails can tear gloves and are difficult to clean properly, especially if they are long. Rings, including wedding rings, can harbor bacteria and cause gloves to tear.

Cleaning and Disinfection

Cleaning is the physical removal of soil, debris, blood, and body fluids from instruments, furniture, and other items. Cleaning is necessary before disinfection because organic debris decreases the effectiveness of disinfectants. Cleaning is an ongoing part of the environmental routing of the clean room environment.

Disinfection is destruction of pathogenic microorganisms by direct exposure to chemical or physical agents. This process is done by using specific detergents that are selected according to the type of instrument to be cleaned. Manufacturer instructions must always be followed for correct dilution, temperature, and use.

Procedure: *Cleaning and Disinfecting*

Objective: To properly clean and disinfect work areas and equipment to prevent the spread of infection.

Equipment Needed: disinfectant, cloth.

Step 1: Thoroughly rinse and/or clean items before a disinfectant is used. The foundation of manual cleaning is friction, which loosens the organic materials and allows their removal during the rinsing process.

Step 2: When cleaning stainless steel instruments, use a back-and-forth motion to follow the grain of the instrument, rather than a circular motion, which can scratch the surface of the item (Figures 7-3A and 7-3B).

Step 3 : To avoid spotting on the instruments, dry the items immediately after rinsing.

Figure 7-3 Proper technique for disinfection. (A) Use back-and-forth motion to cleanse instruments and surfaces (B) Immediately dry and rinse.

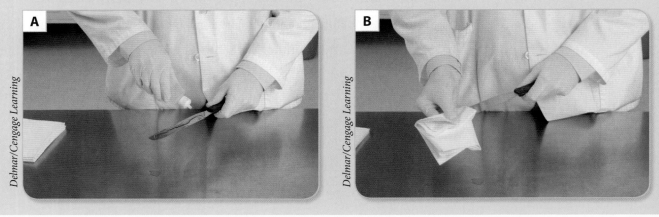

Delmar/Cengage Learning

For surfaces such as countertops, the least expensive and most readil available chemical is a 1:10 solution of ordinary household bleach (**sodiun hypochlorite**).

Exercise

Objective: To become familiar with proper techniques of cleaning and disinfection.

- Properly clean the countertop surface in the laboratory by using correct technique and disinfectants.

- Properly clean and disinfect various stainless steel instruments with the appropriate detergent(s).

Aseptic Technique

The primary method through which microbes are kept to an absolute minimum in the clean room for sterile compounding is aseptic technique. This involves creating a sterile field for each procedure. For sterile compounding in any pharmacy setting, a laminar-airflow hood may be used. Pharmacy technicians must regularly follow the procedures of aseptic technique, which include:

- The removal of all jewelry.

- Not wearing artificial nails because of possible microbial growth around and under them.

- Tying long hair back away from the face.

- Washing hands after entering the work area and before entering a laminar-airflow hood.

- Washing hands, wrists, and arms up to the elbow with warm water and antimicrobial soap for 30 to 90 seconds.

- Putting gloves on, and washing them down with 70% isopropyl alcohol after donning them.

- Washing down the surface of airflow hoods with 70% isopropyl alcohol, following proper procedure.

- Running airflow hoods for at least 30 minutes before beginning work with any medications inside them.

- Not blocking airflow inside a hood at any time with hands or objects.

- Keeping pens and other unneeded objects out of airflow hoods.

- Working at least 6 inches into an airflow hood.

- Avoiding coughing, sneezing, or talking while working inside an airflow hood.

- Wiping down all vials and ports with alcohol.

- Disposing of all needles, syringes, vials, and other byproducts properly.

Alert

When cleaning an airflow hood, do not spray vials and ports with alcohol, because sprayed alcohol can damage an airflow hood's filter.

AUTOCLAVES

Autoclaves are basically pressure cookers that are used to achieve sterilization. They use steam under pressure to obtain temperatures of approximately 250 to 254 °F. Items are exposed to this heat and at least 15 pounds of pressure for specific amounts of time, assuring the killing of all microorganisms and their spores (Figure 7-4). Autoclaves contain

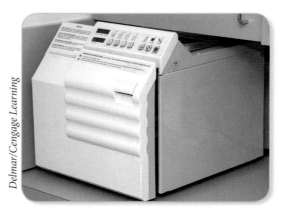

Delmar/Cengage Learning

Figure 7-4 Autoclave.

inner chambers that are surrounded by metal "jackets" that create a middl
steam chamber between the inner sterilizing chamber and the jacket.

They feature a reservoir for distilled water (the only type of wate
that should be used) located inside the jacket. Pharmacy technicians mus
be familiar with the proper operating procedures for autoclaves in th
laboratory. Water is poured into the reservoir and the autoclave's door i
closed and secured. When the autoclave is turned on, the water heats unt
vapor is produced, which enters the middle steam chamber. This pushes th
air in the steam chamber out to increase the pressure, causing the steam t
enter the inner sterilizing chamber where the surgical instruments to b
sterilized have been placed.

The inner chamber pressure then increases, with temperature
reaching their intended peak. The steam reaches all surfaces of each item an
sterilizes them. Unwrapped items are usually sterilized for 20 minutes. Loosel
wrapped items are usually sterilized for 30 minutes, with 40 minutes bein
used for tightly packed items. The pharmacy technician must follow prope
operating procedure for the autoclave to be effective in sterilizing items. Item
to be sterilized must be placed as loosely as possible inside the chamber, with
1- to 3-inch space between packs and walls of the autoclave. Items should no
touch each other in any manner in order to assure complete sterilization.

Autoclaves must be regularly cleaned and maintained. The inne
chamber should be washed with a mild detergent using a cloth that i
rinsed and dried on a daily basis. The outer jacket should be wiped clean
The manufacturer instructions will list the proper methods and material
that should be used. The autoclave should occasionally be drained of wate
and thoroughly cleaned by filling it with a cleaning solution and running i
for a 20-minute cycle. This should be followed by re-emptying it and the
re-filling with distilled rinse water, and another 20-minute cycle. This wate
should be removed following this cycle, with fresh distilled water added fo
its first work cycle after being cleaned. Inner shelves should be removed an

scrubbed. It is important to schedule the cleaning of autoclaves around the work schedules for which they are needed for sterilization. Autoclaves should be inspected during cleaning for any cracking or signs of wear. Replacement rubber seals should be kept on hand in case they need to be changed.

Other items involved in the use of autoclaves include:

- Culture tests – these are strips placed in the center of wrapped articles that are placed into a culture medium after sterilization to check for growth of microorganisms (no growth should occur after proper sterilization); other types of culture testing supplies are also available.

- Sterilization strips – indicators that contain a dye that darkens when exposed to steam at proper temperatures, along with proper pressures and sterilization times; they are placed in the center of wrapped articles (Figures 7-5A and 7-5B).

- Muslin wrap – a cloth wrap used to wrap instruments for sterilization; it may be laundered and reused.

- Paper sterilization wrapping squares – disposable material used instead of muslin wrapping that is used only once and then discarded.

- Sterilization pouches or bags – plastic, paper, or combination-material containers that offer visibility of the items they contain; they are available in different sizes and are commonly used.

- Autoclave tape – chemically treated tape that becomes "striped" when exposed to heat; it is only used to assure that a package has been in a heated autoclave, and not for assurance of full sterilization.

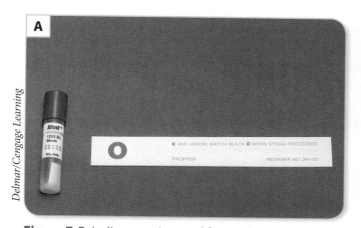

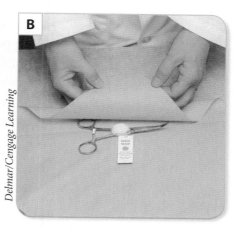

Figure 7-5 Indicator strips used for sterilization.

All items to be sterilized in an autoclave must be labeled clearly with an indelible marker, including the names of the articles, sterilization date, and the initials of the individual who conducted the sterilization. No puncturing or tearing of any packages can be allowed, or the items must be repackaged and re-sterilized. Wrapping techniques must be learned and used according to the laboratory's specific policies and procedures.

CLEAN ROOMS

Clean rooms are specialized work areas (separate rooms) where air quality, humidity, and temperature are highly regulated. This helps to reduce the risk of cross-contamination, and clean room air is filtered repeatedly to remove impurities such as dust particles and particulates. The laminar-airflow hood is located inside the clean room. Most institutional IV rooms are clean rooms and are rated as follows:

- Class 100 – There can be no more than 100 particles larger than 0.5 micron in size in any cubic foot of air.

- Class 1,000 – There can be no more than 1,000 particles larger than 0.5 micron in size in any cubic foot of air.

- Class 10,000 – There can be no more than 10,000 particles larger than 0.5 micron in size in any cubic foot of air.

Clean rooms are usually single-door, positive-pressure rooms designed to keep particulates from flowing into the room when the door is in use. Cardboard items should never be placed in clean rooms because they contain free-floating particles. Positive pressure keeps unfiltered or dirty air from entering, and allows the purified clean room air to offer a reduced risk that contaminants will be introduced into sterile products.

The ceilings, floors, walls, fixtures, counters, cabinets, and shelves located inside clean rooms must all be resistant to sanitizing cleaners. Ceilings that have inlaid panels should be treated with a polymer so that they are hydrophobic and impervious to contaminants. Elastic sealant caulking should be used around the ceiling's perimeter and attached to the supporting frame. Junctures where ceilings and walls meet must be covered or caulked so that there are no recesses or cracks. Ceiling lights should have smooth surfaces, and be mounted flush into the ceiling with appropriate seal material to prevent any gaps or recesses. All other ceiling or wall penetrations must be sealed.

Floors should be made of continuous material with no cracks or breaks, and must be strong and chemically impervious. If possible, floors should have wide vinyl floor coverings that have heat-welded seams extending to the sidewalls. There should not be any sinks or floor drains in the clean room. Walls themselves should be made of hard panels that are connected together with sealing materials. They may also be made of gypsum board that has an epoxy coating or of soft plastic. There should not be any ceiling pipes or other dust-collecting overhangs, and ledges and windowsills should be avoided.

The clean room contains the following major equipment:

- Sterilization devices.

- Laminar-airflow hoods.

- Automated compounding devices.

- Environmental monitoring devices (air particulate counters).

- Clean room garb.

- Cleaning materials.

  - Detergent.

  - Wipers.

  - Sanitizing solutions.

Personal computers, keyboards, monitors, and printers are not allowed inside clean rooms. Printers and paper, for example, add too many tiny particles into the air.

Most of the furniture and equipment found in clean rooms is made of stainless steel, which can be easily cleaned with 70% isopropyl alcohol. Alcohol swabs, needles, and syringes must be kept to a minimum inside clean rooms in order to maintain an aseptic environment.

In January of 2004, the government established USP 797, which greatly improved standards for clean room use and maintenance. All clean room and adjacent anteroom areas must have ceilings, walls, floors, shelving, cabinets, and work surfaces that are free from cracks and crevices, allowing for easy sanitization. There can be no dust-collecting surfaces, and any carts used to transport equipment must be made of stainless steel with high-quality, cleanable casters. See Chapter 9 for further information about USP 797. Figure 7-6 shows an example of a floor plan for clean rooms with adjacent support areas.

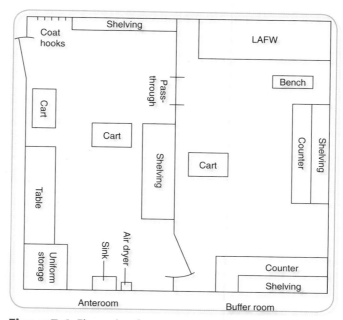

Figure 7-6 Floor plan for anteroom and clean room.

Procedure: *Cleaning Laboratory Furniture with Alcohol*

Objective: To properly perform disinfection and cleaning in the laboratory setting.

Equipment Needed: gloves, cloth, 70% isopropyl alcohol.

Step 1: Don protective gloves before cleaning.

Step 2: Follow policies and procedures to select the correct type of cloth for this purpose.

Step 3: Follow instructions on the 70% isopropyl alcohol container and use the correct amount for each laboratory furniture surface.

Step 4: Avoid touching the cloth to the floor or any potentially hazardous materials, chemicals, or spills.

Step 5: Make sure that the cleaned surfaces are completely dry and are free from residual alcohol before use.

Exercise

Objective: To become familiar with proper techniques of cleaning and disinfection.

Use the steps listed above to practice cleaning laboratory furniture using 70% isopropyl alcohol.

CLEAN AIR ENVIRONMENTS

Parenteral products are regularly prepared in clean room environments. A clean room is described as any specific area that allows no more than 3,500 airborne particles (of no larger than 0.5 microns each) per square meter of air. The United States classifies "clean" or "critical" room environments as "Class 100" or "Grade A." In these environments, the air is rapidly cycled through at rates of approximately 90 to 100 feet per minute.

Incoming air is sent through a pre-filter, then usually treated with an electrostatic unit (that electrically charges particles to remove them by attraction to oppositely charged plates), and then on to a *HEPA* (*high efficiency particulate air*) filter for extremely efficient filtration. Air conditioning and humidity are strictly controlled. A positive air pressure (which is higher than the air pressure outside the clean room) is maintained to prevent outside air from entering through cracks or other openings.

Laminar-Airflow Hoods

Laminar-airflow hoods are designed for the handling of materials whenever sterile working environments are required. These devices use circulating filtered air in parallel flow planes to reduce the risk of bacteria contamination or exposure to chemical pollutants. If operating properly, laminar-airflow hoods are very effective for providing a clean working area. See Figure 7-7 for a depiction of a laminar-airflow hood.

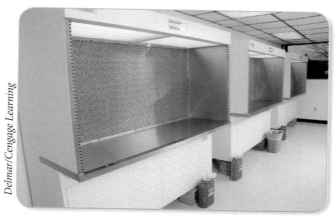

Figure 7-7 Laminar-airflow hood.

Room air may be highly contaminated by normal human actions such as sneezing, which produces up to 200,000 aerosol droplets that can attach to dust particles and remain in the air for weeks. Laminar-airflow hoods are commonly used in pharmacies, surgery areas, laboratories, and food preparation rooms. Laminar-airflow hoods must be certified every 6 months.

Vertical Laminar-Airflow Hoods

There are two types of laminar-airflow hoods: vertical and horizontal. Vertical airflow hoods are used for chemotherapeutic agents because of the direction of airflow and the specifications of the hood. They are also used for mixing non-chemotherapeutic agents. All laminar-airflow hoods basically have a box-like structure, with Plexiglas® tops and sides, and fluorescent lights which illuminate the work area. Positive pressure flowing air (called *laminar*) bathes the work area. This air has passed through a pre-filter to remove lint and dust, and then through a HEPA filter. This type of filter is the most important part of the device, removing very small particles of matter as well as microorganisms. The air is compressed and redistributed into parallel airflow streams, moving at a rate of 90 to 120 linear feet per minute. At this point, there is little to no bacteria remaining in the air. HEPA filters need to be certified every 6 months unless they become wet. HEPA filters must be replaced every 3 to 5 years on average.

Horizontal Laminar-Airflow Hoods

Horizontal airflow hoods are used for the preparation of parenteral medications and sterile product mixtures, and not for chemotherapeutic agents. Figure 7-8 shows both vertical and horizontal airflow hoods and explains their usage.

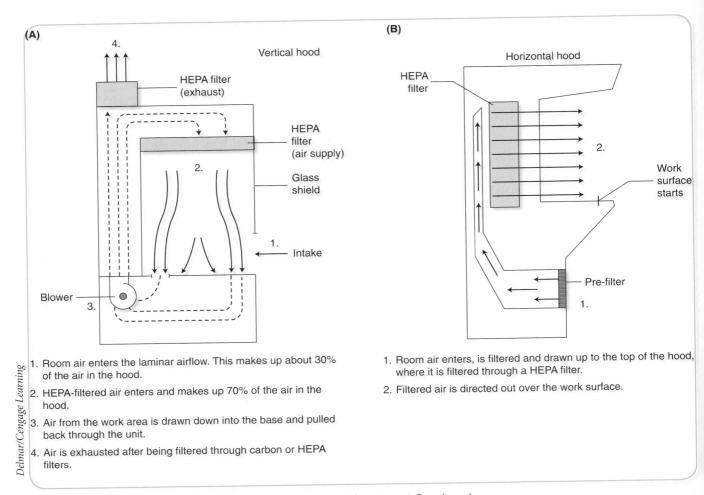

(A)

4.

Vertical hood

HEPA filter
(exhaust)

HEPA
filter
(air supply)

2.

Glass
shield

1.

Intake

Blower

3.

(B)

Horizontal hood

HEPA
filter

2.

Work
surface
starts

Pre-filter

1.

1. Room air enters the laminar airflow. This makes up about 30% of the air in the hood.
2. HEPA-filtered air enters and makes up 70% of the air in the hood.
3. Air from the work area is drawn down into the base and pulled back through the unit.
4. Air is exhausted after being filtered through carbon or HEPA filters.

1. Room air enters, is filtered and drawn up to the top of the hood, where it is filtered through a HEPA filter.
2. Filtered air is directed out over the work surface.

Delmar/Cengage Learning

Figure 7-8 Comparison of a (A) vertical and (B) horizontal laminar-airflow hood.

Horizontal hoods used in hospital pharmacies must be inspected each year by an authorized inspector to ensure the effectiveness of the filtering system. All laminar-airflow hoods should be in limited-access areas with low traffic flow to minimize potential contamination of the hood from the area surrounding it.

Cleaning of Hoods and Clean Rooms

Water and 70% isopropyl alcohol are commonly used for the cleaning of laminar-airflow hoods. Any equipment used for this type of cleaning should be kept in the controlled area and thoroughly cleaned, as well as sanitized, after each use. Hoods must be thoroughly cleaned about every 8 hours or any time they become dirty. Pharmacy technicians who handle compounding should wipe down the hood's surface area when they are done preparing a specific type of compound or product and before they begin compounding another one. The entire procedure for the proper cleaning of hoods is listed below.

Procedure : Cleaning the Laminar-Airflow Hood

Objective: To properly clean the laminar-airflow hood.

Equipment Needed: sterile water, lint-free cloth or gauze, 70% isopropyl alcohol.

Step 1: Wash all hood walls and surfaces with sterile water.

Step 2: Soak any spots that cannot be easily removed for between 5 and 10 minutes, then wipe these spots until they are not visible.

Step 3: Disinfect by wiping all hood surfaces with 70% isopropyl alcohol on a lint-free fabric to reduce lint particles or contaminants, or gauze (when properly done, once this alcohol dries, the hood should be clean).

Step 4: You should wipe from top to bottom on the hood's sides and rear wall (Figures 7-9A and 7-9B).

Step 5: You should wipe from left to right on the flat work surface area (Figure 7-9C).

Step 6: Remember to wipe all parts that are located inside the hood, including the pole and its brackets.

Step 7: The cleaning of the hood must be documented at least every 8 hours, or once every shift.

Figure 7-9 Proper cleaning of a laminar-airflow hood. (A and B) Wipe from top to bottom on sides and rear wall (C) Wipe from left to right on the work surface.

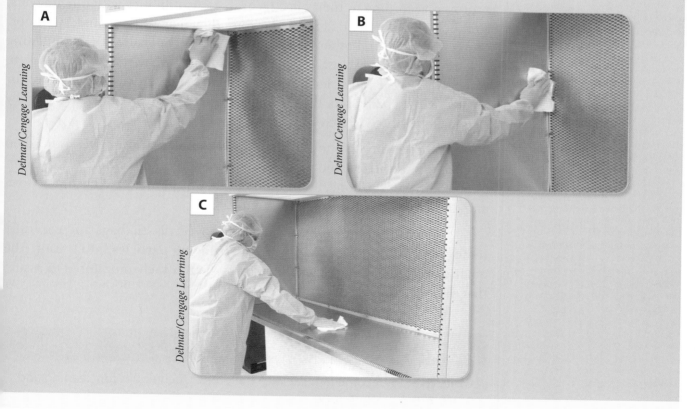

Exercise

Objective: To become familiar with the proper procedure for cleaning the laminar-airflow hood.

Following the steps listed above, demonstrate the proper cleaning of an airflow hood.

Countertops, carts, and any other work surfaces located near the hood should be wiped clean with fresh detergent solution every day. This should be followed with an approved sanitizing agent, allowing sufficient time for its antimicrobial effects to occur. This sanitizing agent should be alternated on a quarterly basis with another agent that exhibits a different type of action. Any spills or other accidents involving contaminating substances must be handled with another cleaning. Ceilings and walls should be cleaned once per month with a mild detergent, followed by an approved sanitizer.

All cleaning and sanitizing agents should be carefully considered and approved according to their effectiveness, compatibilities with other agents, and the types of potentially toxic residues they may leave behind. All mops, sponges, wipers, and other cleaning tools should be made of non-shedding materials and used exclusively in the clean room, followed by the anteroom, and nowhere else. Most cleaning tools should be discarded after one use. For those that may be reused, thorough rinsing and sanitizing must occur. They also must be stored in a clean environment.

Storage shelves should be emptied completely every week and then cleaned and sanitized. Floors should be properly mopped once daily after clean room work is done, but should not be waxed; wax that becomes worn and dried can give off airborne particulates.

Trash should be contained in approved plastic bags and carefully removed from the clean room to avoid bringing particles into the air. The quality of air and surface cleanliness must be routinely monitored to assure that desired quality levels are met.

Exercise

Objective: To become familiar with the proper techniques for cleaning and organizing the laboratory.

Completely empty storage shelves in the laboratory and then properly clean and sanitize them.

In the anteroom area outside a clean room, all supplies and equipment must be sanitized upon being opened. Seventy percent isopropyl alcohol is commonly used along with similar agents for this procedure. This type of alcohol should be filtered through a 0.2-um hydrophobic filter before being used in aseptic areas in order to keep resistant microbial spores from contaminating these areas. Items that are packaged in sealed pouches can be removed from their pouches in the clean room without prior opening and sanitizing, because they are considered already sanitized within their pouches. No cartons used for shipping or packaging should be brought into the clean room.

Anterooms should be properly cleaned and sanitized at least once per week. The floors of anterooms should be properly cleaned and sanitized on a daily basis, working from the section adjoining the clean room outward. Anteroom ceilings and walls should be cleaned and sanitized at least once per quarter. Storage shelves in the anteroom, as well as any refrigerators, should be emptied, cleaned, and sanitized no less than once per month.

SUMMARY

Aseptic technique is of the utmost importance in eliminating microorganisms and avoiding contamination during sterile compounding. The safety of the patient and the control of infection are the main aims of sterile compounding. Aseptic compounding is practiced on products prepared in an institutional setting, a home infusion pharmacy, or a pharmaceutical manufacturing facility. The principles are the same, but the practices differ.

Among different types of microorganisms, bacteria and viruses are of the most concern related to the practice of aseptic technique during sterile compounding. The sources of contamination can be divided into two groups: environmental and endogenous. Environmental sources include personnel, environment, and contaminated instruments.

Medical asepsis practices are based on hand washing, general cleaning, and disinfecting of contaminated surfaces. For sterile compounding of pharmaceutical agents, there are specialized work areas where air quality, humidity, and temperature are highly regulated. This helps to reduce the risk of cross-contamination, and clean room air is filtered repeatedly to remove impurities such as dust particles and particulates.

Laminar-airflow hoods are designed for handling of materials whenever sterile working environments are required. These devices use circulating filtered air in parallel flow planes to reduce the risk of bacterial contamination or exposure to chemical pollutants.

REVIEW QUESTIONS

Multiple Choice

1. High-efficiency particulate airflow (HEPA) filters must be certified every:

    A. 2 months
    B. 4 months
    C. 6 months
    D. 2 years

2. How long must the blower run in a laminar-airflow hood prior to use?

    A. 5 minutes
    B. 15 minutes
    C. 30 minutes
    D. 45 minutes

3. The smallest microorganisms include which of the following?

    A. bacteria
    B. fungi
    C. viruses
    D. protozoa

4. Which of the following types of environments should a laminar-airflow hood provide?

   A. Class 100,000 area   C. Class 1,000 area
   B. Class 10,000 area   D. Class 100 area

5. The physical removal of soil, debris, and body fluids from instruments, furniture, or other items, is referred to as:

   A. cleaning   C. sterilization
   B. disinfection   D. none of the above

6. Which of the following factors play a great role in defending against infections?

   A. a host's cardiovascular system
   B. a host's integumentary system
   C. a host's immune system
   D. a host's respiratory system

7. Most institutional intravenous clean rooms are rated as:

   A. Class 10,000   C. Class 100
   B. Class 1,000   D. all of the above

8. Cardboard items should never be placed in clean rooms because they contain:

   A. pathogens   C. asbestos
   B. free-floating particles   D. A and B

9. Most of the furniture inside clean rooms should be cleaned with which of the following?

   A. 10% bleach
   B. 20% isopropyl alcohol
   C. 70% isopropyl alcohol
   D. 100% isopropyl alcohol

10. The United States classifies "clean" or "critical" room environments as "Class 100" or:

    A. "Grade A"   C. "Grade C"
    B. "Grade B"   D. "Grade D"

Fill in the Blank

1. The process of inhibiting the growth and multiplication of microorganisms is referred to as _____.

2. A large part of compounding awareness concerns proper _____ and the proper wearing of intact gloves to prevent skin contamination.

3. Medical asepsis is the use of practices such as hand washing, _____, and _____ of contaminated surfaces.

4. The hands can usually be washed effectively in 15 to 20 _____.

5. Most of the furniture found in clean rooms is made of _____, which can be easily cleaned with 70% isopropyl alcohol.

6. The United States classifies "clean" or "critical" room environments as "Class 100" or "_____."

7. Vertical airflow hoods are used for _____ agents because of the direction of airflow and the specifications of the hood.

8. Horizontal airflow hoods are used for the preparation of _____ medications and sterile product mixtures.

9. Horizontal hoods used in hospital pharmacies must be inspected each _____ by an authorized inspector.

10. Hoods must be thoroughly cleaned about every _____ or any time they become _____.

CHAPTER 8

Equipment, Garments, and Gowning

OUTLINE

Equipment

Syringes

Needles

Ampules

Vials

Filters

Intravenous Tubing

Vented Tubing

Intravenous Bags

Dispensing Pins

Port Adapters

Vented Spike Adapters

Auxiliary Labels

Sharps Containers

Refrigerators

Freezers

Computer Terminals and Software

Carts

Locker Facilities

Miscellaneous Equipment

Balances

Warming Cabinets

Microwave Ovens

OBJECTIVES

Upon completion of this chapter, the student should be able to:

1. Describe the equipment used in sterile compounding procedures.
2. Differentiate between Viaflex bags and dark bags.
3. Demonstrate the proper techniques for gloving, masking, and gowning during sterile compounding.
4. Explain the purpose of using sharps containers.
5. Differentiate between ampules and vials.
6. Describe the characteristics of special refrigerators in the sterile compounding pharmacy.
7. Explain the purpose of auxiliary labels.

GLOSSARY

Ampule – A small glass container commonly used to hold hypodermic injection solutions or powders for reconstitution into these solutions; they often have tops that are designed to easily break off prior to use.

Carts – Vehicles commonly used to move supplies and equipment in medical workplaces.

Filter – A device used to separate certain elements or particles from a solution.

Gauge – The size of the needle.

Intravenous (IV) bags – Pre-filled, sterile plastic bags used to contain intravenous solutions prior to administration.

Intravenous (IV) tubing – Plastic tubing used to transfer intravenous fluids from IV bags or bottles, through needles, into the body.

Needles – Hollow devices commonly used to inject medications into the body, or to withdraw fluids from the body.

Sharps – Any sharp medical equipment, including needles, catheters, and other equipment that may potentially cause injury during handling.

Syringes – The parts of hypodermic needle assemblies used to contain medications prior to injection through the actual needle into the body, or to contain fluids withdrawn from the body.

Vials – Small glass bottles that are commonly sealed with rubber or cork stoppers and used to store medications prior to use.

OVERVIEW

Most sterile compounding occurs in the hospital and home health care environments. During sterile compounding there is a need for clean air environments. Final compounded products must be free from physical or chemical contaminants as well as from microorganisms. Sterilization is also an essential concept in the preparation of sterile pharmaceutical products. Its aim is to provide products that are safe and to eliminate the possibility of introducing infection.

Pharmacy technicians must be familiar with equipment, devices, clean air environments, garments, and gowning for the processes involved in sterile compounding.

EQUIPMENT

There are many tools and devices that are required for compounding sterile preparations. These tools and devices includes the items listed below.

Syringes

Disposable **syringes** are sterilized, prepackaged, nonpyrogenic (not causing fever), nontoxic, and ready to use. They are available in a variety of sizes that range from less than 1 mL to over 60 mL. These syringes have marked cylinders (or barrels) to assist in measuring doses accurately. The component parts of a syringe consist of a plunger, barrel, flange, and tip (Figure 8-1).

- The *plunger* is a movable cylinder designed for insertion within the barrel; it provides the mechanism by which a medication (or other substance) is drawn into or pushed out of the barrel.

- The *barrel* is the part that holds the medication and has graduated markings (calibrations) on its surface for use in measuring medications.

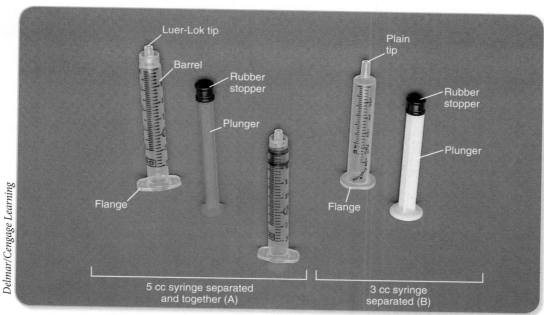

Delmar/Cengage Learning

Figure 8-1 Parts of a syringe.

Alert

Common sizes of syringes that are used for sterile compounding are: 1 mL, 3 mL, 6mL, 12 mL, 20 mL, 35 mL, and 60 mL.

- The *flange* is at the end of the barrel where the plunger is inserted. It forms a rim around the end of the barrel where the plunger is inserted and has appendages against which one places the index and middle fingers when drawing up solution for injection. The flange also prevents the syringe from rolling when laid on a flat surface.

- The *tip* is at the end of the barrel where the needle is attached.

Exercise

Objective: To become familiar with the parts of a needle and syringe and how they function.

Demonstrate and describe the parts of a syringe and a needle. Practice drawing up specific amounts of liquid into the syringe.

Alert

Pharmacy technicians must ensure that the syringe tip, the inside of the barrel, the shaft and rubber plunger tip, and the shaft of the needle are all kept sterile.

The pharmacy technician should only touch the outside of the barrel and the plunger's handle. The parts of a syringe must remain sterile during the preparation, compounding, and administration of parenteral medications that are inside the barrel.

Procedure: *Opening a Prepackaged Syringe*

Objective: To properly open a syringe and maintain sterility of the product.

Equipment Needed: prepackaged syringe, gloves

Step 1: Wash your hands.

Step 2: Choose the correct syringe for the required procedure—this depends upon the amount of medication needed.

Step 3: Put on protective gloves.

Step 4: Pull apart the top ends of the packaging, using a separating motion, moving the hands away from each other.

Step 5: Withdraw the prepackaged syringe assembly.

Alert

- *Used needles and syringes should be discarded in a rigid, puncture-proof container.*

- *Do not recap a needle after giving an injection. Most needle sticks occur while recapping. Refer to Chapter 1 for OSHA regulations.*

Needles

Most **needles** are disposable, made of stainless steel, and individually packaged for sterility. The needle has three basic parts: the hub (which fits onto the syringe); the shaft (which is attached to the hub); and the bevel (which is the slanted part at the tip of the shaft). Needles come in various lengths, ranging from ¼ inch to 3 inches, with gauges that range from 28 to 14 (Figures 8-2A and 8-2B).

The **gauge** of a needle refers to the diameter of its shaft. The larger the gauge number, the smaller the diameter of the shaft.

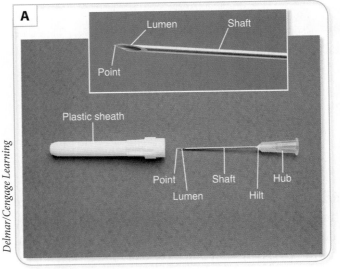

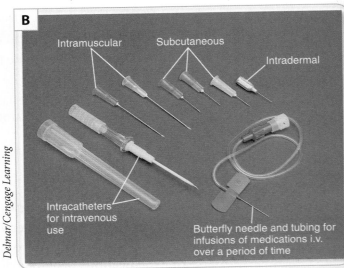

Figure 8-2 Sizes and types of needles (different colored hubs denote needle gauges).

Procedure: Attaching a Needle to a Syringe

Objective: To properly prepare a syringe by attaching a needle to it.

Equipment Needed: syringe, needle

Step 1: Wash your hands.

Step 2: Choose the proper size needle and syringe for the required procedure.

Step 3: If the needle is paper-covered, peel apart the package so that the needle hub is exposed.

Step 4: If the needle is plastic-covered, twist off the end that covers the hub.

Step 5: Hold the needle, still in its protective packaging, in one hand while holding the syringe in the other hand (Figure 8-3).

Step 6: If the syringe has a luer-lock attachment, gently twist the syringe counter clockwise while pushing it toward the needle (you will feel it tighten once it is attached).

Step 7: If the syringe has a tapered (or "slip-fit") attachment, simply push the needle onto the syringe until they are tightly attached together.

Step 8: Remove all of the needle packaging and dispose of it properly.

Step 9: The assembled needle and syringe are ready to be used.

Figure 8-3 Attach needle to syringe.

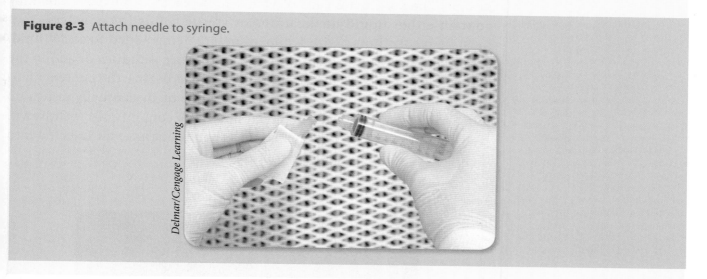

Delmar/Cengage Learning

Alert

Always remember to keep your fingers away from the point of attachment when attaching a needle to a syringe.

Ampules

An **ampule** is a small, sterile, pre-filled glass container that usually holds a single dose of a hypodermic solution (Figure 8-4). Most ampules have a constriction in the stem, marked with a colored band, to facilitate opening the ampule. They contain sterile medicinal solutions or powders to be made up into solutions and used for injection or for sterile compounding solutions. Contents of ampules should be withdrawn with filter needles or straws, which are removed and replaced with a regular needle before injecting the drug into the desired solution. Ampules themselves have a 5-micron filter designed to remove particles that may fall into them upon opening.

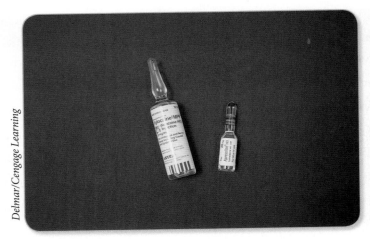

Delmar/Cengage Learning

Figure 8-4 Ampules.

Vials

Vials are small, sterile, pre-filled glass bottles with soft metal or rubber caps (Figure 8-5). They are either single- or multiple-dose in design. The soft metal caps of vials can be easily removed. Vials may contain either liquid medications or sterile solids (or powders) that must be reconstituted with a diluent before being added to an IV fluid. A needle is inserted through the stopper to either withdraw or add to the contents. Excessive air forced into a vial can aerosolize the contents into the air or even burst the vial. An equal volume of air is usually drawn up in a syringe and injected into a vial before its contents are withdrawn. However, pressurized vial medications should not have air injected into them before withdrawal of the contents.

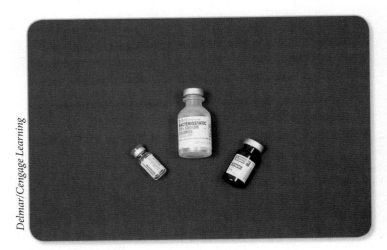

Delmar/Cengage Learning

Figure 8-5 Vials.

Procedure: Withdrawing a Solution from a Vial

Objective: To demonstrate the proper procedure for withdrawing a solution from a vial.

Equipment Needed: solution, syringe and needle, vial, gloves, alcohol wipe, needle cover

Step 1: Assemble all required equipment and materials.

Step 2: Wash your hands.

Step 3: Verify that the vial you select contains the proper type and amount of required medication.

Step 4: Choose the correct needle and syringe (assemble if necessary, or open a prepackaged needle and syringe, leaving the needle cap on).

Step 5: Put on gloves.

Step 6: Compare the drug order and the vial for verification.

Step 7: Roll the vial between your palms. This agitates the medication and mixes any settled particles back into the solution.

Step 8: Visibly inspect the medication for clarity.

Step 9: Verify that the medication has not reached its expiration date (Figure 8-6A).

Step 10: Using an alcohol wipe, clean the vial's rubber stopper with a circular motion (Figure 8-6B).

Step 11: Place the vial on a flat surface and leave the alcohol swab over the vial's rubber stopper.

Step 12: Pick up the syringe and draw up air by grasping the plunger. Make sure the amount you draw up is exactly the amount of medication required (Figure 8-6C).

Step 13: Insert the needle into the cover of the vial's rubber stopper while the vial is still on a flat surface. Do not touch the needle to anything except the clean rubber stopper (Figure 8-6D).

Step 14: Inject the drawn-up air into the vial from the syringe.

Step 15: Pick up the syringe and vial while keeping them together and turn them so that the vial is upside down above the syringe (Figure 8-6E).

Step 16: Slowly withdraw, at eye level, the proper amount of medication from the vial (Figure 8-6F).

Step 17: Check that there are no air bubbles in the syringe.

Step 18: If there are air bubbles, use one hand to grasp the vial and syringe together. Use your other hand to tap the syringe until the air bubbles dislodge and are transferred into the syringe's tip.

Step 19: Gently expel these air bubbles through the needle.

Step 20: Continue withdrawing medication until the required amount is in the syringe, with no air bubbles.

Step 21: Withdraw the needle from the vial.

Step 22: Replace the needle cover without allowing the needle to touch anywhere except the inside of the needle cover.

Step 23: Verify that you have the correct drug and dosage.

Step 24: Return the medication vial to the proper shelf or refrigerator.

Step 25: The syringe is now ready for use.

Procedure: (Continued)

Figure 8-6 Removing medication from a vial. (A) Check the expiration date (B) Swab the top of the vial with alcohol (C) Draw air into syringe (D) Insert syringe into vial (E) Inject air into the vial (F) Withdraw fluid from vial.

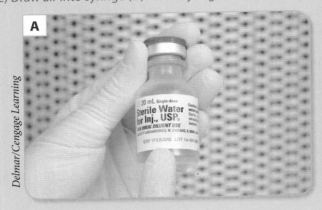

A

Delmar/Cengage Learning

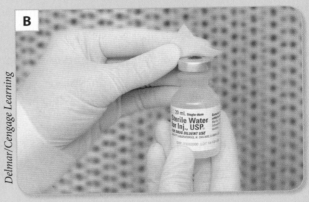

B

Delmar/Cengage Learning

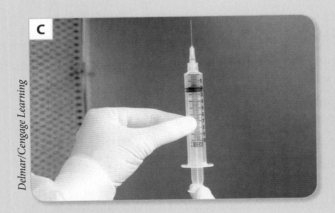

C

Delmar/Cengage Learning

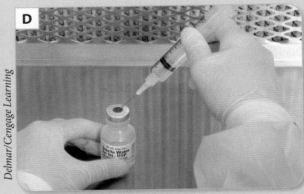

D

Delmar/Cengage Learning

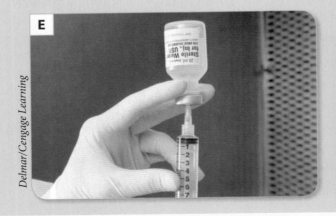

E

Delmar/Cengage Learning

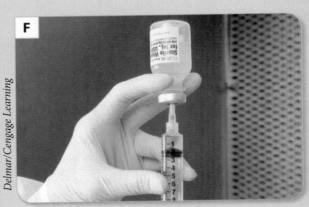

F

Delmar/Cengage Learning

Filters

A **filter** is a device or material through which a gas or liquid passes in order to separate out unwanted matter (Figure 8-7). Filters are made of various types of porous materials, through which liquids or gasses are passed to separate them from contained particulate matter or impurities. They are used to eliminate air, bacteria, fungi, and particulates from solutions as well.

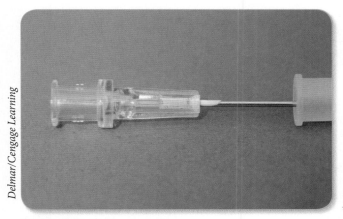

Delmar/Cengage Learning

Figure 8-7 Filtered needle.

Exercise: Using filters

Objective: To properly use a filter to separate particles from a substance.

Use a filter placed across a funnel by pouring a liquid through it to remove any suspended particles. Practice by using a cup of coffee to remove any grounds.

Intravenous Tubing

Intravenous (IV) tubing is available in different subcategories, which include primary, extension, and secondary (or piggyback) sets. Extension sets are used close to a patient's IV site, and can be one piece of tubing, divided into two parts, or divided into three parts. Extension sets are usually between 3 and 55 inches in length. Secondary sets are used with primary sets, usually connected to a Y-site on the primary line. They measure between 20 and 45 inches in length. Primary IV sets are explained below.

Primary IV Tubing

IV therapy is performed by a physician or a registered nurse, who will insert a needle or catheter into an appropriate vein and attach tubing to the catheter. The tubing is inserted into a glass or plastic container of fluid. Primary IV tubing sets are sometimes called "administration sets." A sterile dressing covers the skin surrounding the IV site. Primary IV tubing is usually 60 inches or longer, and can be used with IV pumps (which are electronic devices) or by itself for gravity infusions (Figure 8-8). Electronic devices for infusion are mechanisms powered by batteries, electricity, or a combination of both. These devices are safe and precise, and can be programmed to infuse at a specific rate. They can signal when the infusion is complete. These devices have alarms that alert the health care provider if there is a problem with air in the system or pressure in the line (see Figure 8-9).

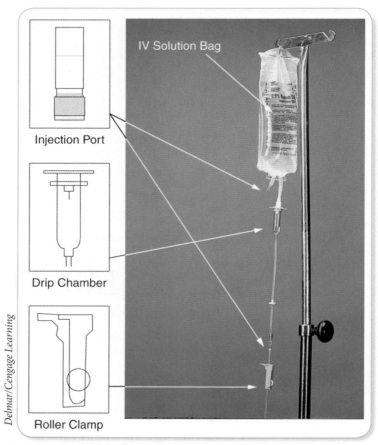

Figure 8-8 IV administration set.

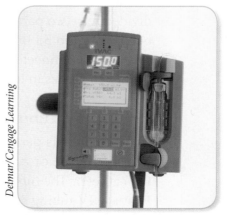

Figure 8-9 Infusion pump.
(Courtesy of Alaris Medical Systems.)

Vented Tubing

This type of tubing is primarily used to transfer fluids from one container to another so that it can be administered to a patient. Only one solution can be transferred at a given time (see Figure 8-10).

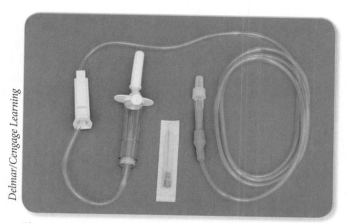

Figure 8-10 Vented IV set.

Intravenous Bags

Intravenous (IV) bags are usually made of plastic and have an attached drip container that allows the fluid they contain to flow one drop at a time. When used for a gravity drip, they are placed above the level of the patient. Common fluids administered from IV bags include sodium chloride, dextrose, lactated Ringer's solution, acetic acid, and sterile water.

Viaflex Bags

These IV bags are commonly used in many medical environments, being constructed of PVC (polyvinyl chloride) plastic, with no latex. They are very resistant to breakage, easy to handle, and inexpensive. They are commonly available in 250 to 2000 mL sizes, though others are available (Figure 8-11).

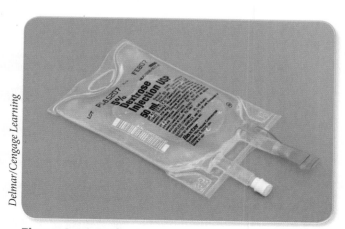

Figure 8-11 Viaflex bags.

Alert

Piggyback IVs are commonly used for admixtures of antibiotics and contain less than 100 mL of solution.

Empty Evacuated Containers

These glass containers use vacuum (or negative pressure) to safely hold a variety of solutions. Rubber stoppers on the top help to seal them from outside contamination. They are available in a variety of sizes, and can be easily heated in an autoclave if required.

Dark Bags

For medications that must be kept away from direct light, dark bags are used. These bags are amber in color, and can easily be placed over a variety of different containers (including bottles, syringes, and IV sets) to protect from light contamination.

Dispensing Pins

These vented pins allow easy transferring of fluids from vials to wherever they are needed. They use a luer-lock system, which locks a needle onto a syringe's nozzle.

Port Adapters

These adapters are "male" adapters, used to attach to the IV additive port of an IV bag. By using port adapters for most needle sticks, only one needle stick needs to occur in the IV additive port.

Vented Spike Adapters

These adapters are primarily made of plastic, and are used in the venting of glass bottles which are attached to IV tubing. They are also available in a high-speed design.

Auxiliary Labels

Auxiliary labels include instructional labels that help in the correct storage of medications. Auxiliary labels may include a wide variety of instructions such as "do not refrigerate," "keep refrigerated," or "protect from light" (Figure 8-12).

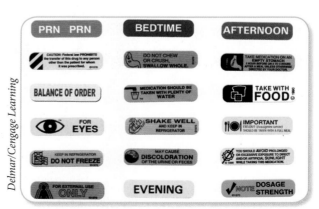

Delmar/Cengage Learning

Figure 8-12 Auxiliary labels.

Sharps Containers

These containers are required to be used for the disposal of any glass equipment (such as broken bottles, used vials, etc.), needles, syringes, and blood-related products. Some **sharps** containers are specially colored, such as red sharps containers, which require controlled and authorized disposal (Figure 8-13).

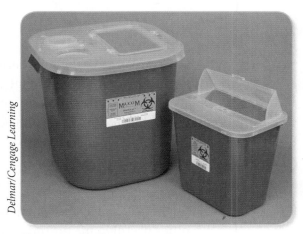

Figure 8-13 Sharps container.

Refrigerators

Special refrigerators used in medicine are designed to feature strengthened doors, heat-treated finishes, and hospital-grade electrical plugs. They have commercial-grade fan motors, condensers, and compressors to ensure long-term, energy-efficient operation. Refrigerators in the compounding pharmacy should bear alert signs stating that no food or drinks should be stored inside them.

Freezers

Special freezers used in medicine are similar to the designs of medical refrigerators, but maintain much colder temperatures to allow for complete freezing of most materials.

Computer Terminals and Software

Most sterile preparation programs use special computer software at dedicated terminals in specific areas away from the sterile preparation area. There are many commercially available software programs specifically designed for this usage.

Alert

A printer located in the anteroom is connected with the computer system and can print out labels for compounding.

Exercise

Objective: To become familiar with computer software and programs.

Use the computer software that is available in your workplace and print 3 sterile preparation orders for compounding.

Carts

Heavy-duty stainless steel **carts** are preferred for moving components an final preparations of solutions. They feature 6-inch swiveling wheels, brake and heavy wire mesh shelving. Cardboard boxes should never be place on these carts in order to avoid contamination of the sterile preparatio area. Sometimes, smaller stainless steel carts are used for moving materia directly into critical areas.

Locker Facilities

These areas are used for changing into sterile gowns, gloves, masks, et Most locker facilities of this type have lockable storage containers, sinks wit floor controls, and soap dispensers for hand washing. These locker faciliti should be located as close to the controlled area as possible.

MISCELLANEOUS EQUIPMENT

Balances (scales), special microwave ovens, and warming storage cabine are other useful items for the preparation of sterile medications.

Balances

Balances are scales that are used for measuring different component such as compounding powders that may be needed for a preparation.

Warming Cabinets

These cabinets store and warm certain drugs that may be prone t crystallization, such as mannitol.

Microwave Ovens

Specialized microwave ovens with digital readouts may be required t assist in warming certain substances used in sterilized preparations.

GARMENTS

Garments (sometimes referred to as "garb") should be appropriate fc the types of preparations being compounded. The way they are constructe and their barrier properties are important in keeping out harmful material Seams of all garments should be contained and closures must be taut the neck, ankles, and wrists. Garment fabrics must provide a barrier fc very small particles, must not shed particles, and must be able to dissipat electrostatic charges. Non-woven garment materials such as Tyvek ar preferred because, though they may only be used once, they provide bette protection from hazardous materials.

Gowns

A gown made of a moisture-resistant material is used when working with blood, body fluids, or other chemical substances. The gown prevents contamination by soiling or splashing of fluids, keeping these fluids away from the health care provider's uniform. Gowns (as well as "coveralls") should be made of material that protects against the passage of bacteria and drugs. The fabric should be woven sufficiently to achieve a reasonable barrier, without making the wearer feel excessively warm. Newer gowning materials provide good protection, improved appearance, and enough air permeability to allow for the comfort of the wearer. These outfits can be washed in high-temperature water, and be exposed to chlorine, steam autoclaves, ethylene oxide, and radiation as used for sterilization. Gowns should be discarded according to facility policy after use.

Procedure: Donning a Gown

Objective: To properly demonstrate the donning of a gown to protect oneself from infectious or hazardous materials.

Equipment Needed: gown

Step 1: Wash hands thoroughly and dry completely.

Step 2: Grasp the center of the gown near the neck, avoiding touching its wrapper (Figure 8-14A).

Step 3: Lift the gown while keeping away from any equipment (Figure 8-14B).

Step 4: Determine the inside and outside portions of the gown.

Step 5: Hold the gown near the shoulders and let it unfold (Figure 8-14C).

Step 6: Position the gown so that the arms may be easily slipped inside (Figure 8-14D).

Step 7: Slip the gown over your arms, keeping your hands within the cuffs (Figure 8-14E).

Step 8: Flex your arms and elbows to hold the gown in place (Figure 8-14F).

Step 9: Have an assistant adjust the gown and secure the neck and back properly.

Figure 8-14 Donning a gown. (A) Pick gown up by center without touching sterile packaging (B) Lift gown away from packaging and keep from touching any other items.

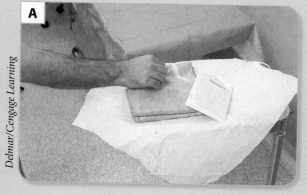
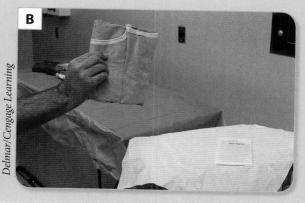

Delmar/Cengage Learning

Procedure: (Continued)

Figure 8-14 Donning a gown. (C) Allow gown to unfold (D) Position gown so that you are able to slide your arms into it. (E) Slide arms into gown without putting hands through cuffs (F) Allow assistant to secure gown in back.

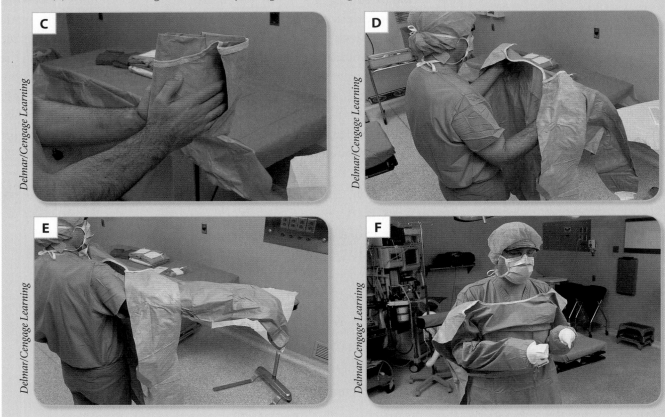

More information about gowning and gowning techniques is give later in this chapter.

Gloves

The use of gloves prevents the spread of disease. Usually, pharmac technicians will wear nonsterile latex or vinyl disposable gloves for nonsteril compounding, and sterile gloves when sterile compounding procedures a required.

Pharmacy technicians should also wear gloves if they have cuts open sores on their hands. Gloves may be used during many routine cleanin procedures performed by the pharmacy technician. Utility gloves may b worn for certain cleaning procedures. The use of gloves does not replac the need for hand washing. Always wash the hands before and after glov use. Upon accidentally touching a potentially contaminated environment surface after removing gloves, wash the hands again.

Alert

The gloves are removed to open doors, turn on faucets, or touch other environmental surfaces and supplies.

For gloves to be effective, they must be intact and have no visible cuts, tears, or cracks. They must fit the hands well. Gloves come in different sizes. Do not wash the hands while wearing gloves. Hand washing damages the pores of the gloves and may allow microbes to enter.

Procedure: Donning Gloves

Objective: To demonstrate the proper method of donning gloves to practice infection control techniques.

Equipment Needed: gloves

Step 1: Select a pair of sterile gloves.

Step 2: Remove the first glove from the packaging, keeping your fingers within the cuff of the gown (Figure 8-15A).

Step 3: Place the glove on the palm of your hand with the thumb side of the glove toward your palm (Figure 8-15B).

Step 4: Pull the glove's cuff over the cuff of the gown.

Step 5: Unfold the glove's cuff so that it completely covers the cuff of the gown.

Step 6: Grasp both the glove and gown at the level of the wrist.

Step 7: As you pull the glove into position, work your fingers into the glove.

Step 8: Repeat the above steps for the second glove (Figures 8-15C).

Figure 8-15 Donning gloves. (A) Keeping hand in cuff of gown, remove glove from package (B) Position glove with fingers facing toward arm (C) Pull glove on and adjust.

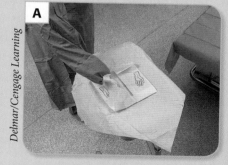
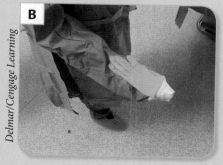
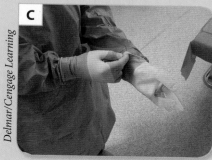

Delmar/Cengage Learning

Procedure: Proper Removal and Disposal of Gloves

Objective: To demonstrate proper removal of gloves to prevent contamination and infection of hazardous materials.

Equipment Needed: gloves, gown, biohazard container

Step 1: Use your dominant hand to grasp the glove of the opposite hand near the palm. Your arms should be extended from your body, with your hands pointed down.

Step 2: Pull the glove inside out until you reach your fingers, holding the glove inside your dominant, gloved hand.

Step 3: Insert the thumb of your non-gloved hand inside the cuff of the remaining glove.

Step 4: Pull the glove down, inside out, over the first removed glove. This leaves the contaminated side of both gloves on the inside.

Step 5: Dispose of the gloves together in a biohazard waste container.

Step 6: Wash your hands.

Face Masks

Face masks should be worn when exposure to droplet secretions ma[y] occur. These masks should cover the pharmacy technician's nose and mout[h] (Figure 8-16). The mask should be tied to fit snugly, using either the elasti[c] band or strings that are attached to the mask. If the mask has strings, mak[e] sure that they do not cross each other when they are tied behind the hea[d.] This will ensure a snug fit. Just prior to working in a horizontal laminar airflow workbench, masks should be put on. They are for optional use whe[n] working in vertical workbenches or other equipment that has solid barrier[s] between the operator's face and the workspace. Masks should be replaced [if] they get wet, as dampness decreases their protection level. They should als[o] be replaced each time a worker leaves the compounding area, or wheneve[r] their integrity of cleanliness may be compromised.

Alert

Masks are commonly worn to filter moisture that may be expelled from the mouth and nasopharynx due to normal breathing, talking, sneezing, or coughing.

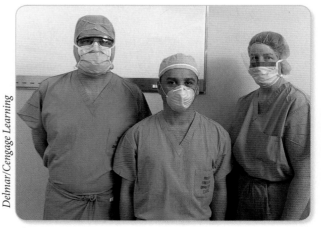

Delmar/Cengage Learning

Figure 8-16 Face masks.

Procedure: Proper Donning of Face Masks

Objective: To demonstrate the proper procedure for donning a mask to prevent contamination from hazardous substances.

Equipment Needed: mask

Step 1: Wash your hands.

Step 2: Place the mask so that it covers your nose, mouth, and chin.

Step 3: Fit the flexible nose piece over the bridge of your nose.

Step 4: Secure around your head (whether it has ties or elastic).

Step 5: Adjust so that it fits comfortably.

Alert

After use, masks should be removed and discarded into proper waste containers.

Shoe Covers

Shoe covers should be put on before the wearer's shoes touch the floor on the clean side of a workspace or the wearer crosses a specially marked area of the floor. Slip-on shoe covers are commonly used, but for some high-risk compounding, ankle-length "booties" are preferred to provide complete coverage between the cuffs of pants and the shoes (Figure 8-17).

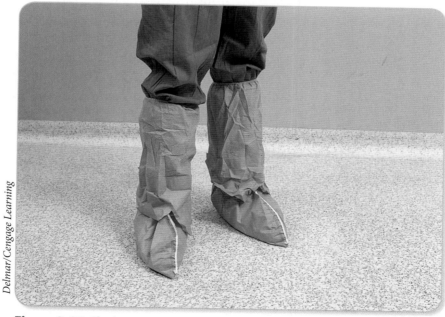

Delmar/Cengage Learning

Figure 8-17 Shoe covers.

Procedure: *Proper Donning of Shoe Covers*

Objective: To demonstrate the proper method of donning shoe covers.

Equipment Needed: shoe covers

Step 1: If the shoe cover is of the type that only covers the actual footwear, simply slip each of them over your footwear so that the elastic band encircles the top.

Step 2: If the shoe cover is of the "boot" type, simply pull them over your footwear and up to just below the knees, allowing the elastic to secure itself at this point.

GOWNING

Gowning should be selected based on the types of preparations to b compounded and the cleanliness level in the compounding area. Clothing that produces lint should be avoided. Risk 1 Level garb consists of usuall a clean gown or closed coat with elastic sleeve cuffs. Masks, hair, and facial hair covers should be worn. Hands and arms should be scrubbed appropriately with approved cleansers. Risk 2 Level garb includes all of the Risk 1 requirements, plus gloves and shoe covers. Risk 3 Level garb include full clean-room attire, consisting of low-shedding coveralls, head covers face masks, shoe covers, and sterile gloves.

Gowning Techniques

Gowning normally takes place in an area that is equipped for hand washing, as well as for the storage of personal clothes and clean-room garments. Employees should walk over an adhesive mat designed to loosen particles from their shoes before entering the gowning area. They should then store their outer personal garments, and put on scrubs or other appropriate uniforms. Employees should remove all jewelry and makeup, and thoroughly wash their hands before putting on clean-room garments. They should dry their hands and arms with lint-free towels.

In most cases, clean-room gowning is put on from the head down, a follows:

- Head covers or hoods.

- Face masks and/or beard covers.

- Protective eyewear.

- Gowns, closed coats, or coveralls.

- Shoe covers, over-boots, or second pairs of shoe covers.
- Gloves.

Exercise

Objective: To become familiar with the proper order and procedures for donning PPE.

Practice donning a face mask, protective eyewear, a gown, shoe covers, and gloves in the proper order and manner.

SUMMARY

Common equipment used for sterile compounding includes disposable syringes and needles, glass ampules, rubber-capped vials, porous filters, IV tubing, IV bags of different types, dark bags, evacuated containers, and a variety of adaptive equipment that allow easier compounding operations. Auxiliary equipment includes labels, sharps containers, cooling and heating devices, computer systems, carts, locker facilities, and balances.

Other equipment includes garments such as gowns, masks, protective eyewear, and shoe covers. Proper gowning techniques protect the compounding environment and allow the correct garments to be effectively used for the performance of sterile compounding.

REVIEW QUESTIONS

Multiple Choice

1. Which of the following parts of a needle refers to the diameter of its shaft?

   A. hub

   B. tip

   C. bevel

   D. gauge

2. Which of the following parts of a syringe holds the medication and has graduated markings?

   A. plunger

   B. tip

   C. flange

   D. barrel

3. Intravenous tubing is available in different subcategories. Which of the following sets is *not* included?

   A. spike adapter

   B. extension

   C. primary

   D. piggyback

4. Which of the following is an advantage of Viaflex bags?

   A. they are inexpensive

   B. they are very resistant to breakage

   C. they are easy to handle

   D. all of the above

5. Which of the following is used to attach to the IV additive post of an IV bag?

   A. spike adapter

   B. male adapter

   C. vented adapter

   D. female adapter

Matching

1. _____ Fits onto the syringe
2. _____ Designed for insertion within the barrel
3. _____ Holds the medication and has calibrations
4. _____ Forms a rim around the end of the barrel
5. _____ Where the needle is attached

   A. Flange
   B. Tip
   C. Plunger
   D. Barrel
   E. Hub

Fill in the Blank

1. Needles come in various lengths, ranging from _____ inch to _____ inches.

2. Secondary IV tubing sets are used with primary sets, and usually to a Y-site on the _____.

3. Vented tubing is primarily used to transfer _____ from one container to _____.

4. Dispensing pins use a _____ system, which locks a needle onto a syringe's nozzle.

5. Port adapters are "_____" adapters, used to attach to the IV additive post of an IV bag.

6. Instructional labels that help in the correct storage of medications are called _____ labels.

7. Garment fabrics must provide a barrier for very small _____ and must not shed particles.

8. Masks should be replaced if they get _____, and they should also be replaced each time a technician leaves the compounding _____.

9. Gowning usually occurs in a room outside the _____ area.

10. Pharmacy technicians must remove all jewelry and makeup, and thoroughly wash their hands before putting on clean-room _____.

SOURCE

http://www.pharmacists.ca/content/hcp/Resource_Centre/ Practice_Resources/pdf/chapter.pdf

Sterile Preparations and Procedures of Compounding

OBJECTIVES

Upon completion of this chapter, the student should be able to:

1. Define a sterile product.
2. Explain the concept of laminar-airflow.
3. Describe non-injectable products.
4. Explain factors affecting parenteral products.
5. Outline the major categories of parenteral drugs.
6. Explain piggyback and IV push.
7. Define the technician's role in parenteral admixtures.
8. Demonstrate the proper procedures for preparing parenteral admixtures.

GLOSSARY

Aseptic technique – Preparing and handling sterile products in a manner that prevents microbial contamination.

Beyond-use date – A date for a sterile drug product calculated from the time it is compounded until it is administered to a patient.

Conjunctiva – A thin, clear, moist membrane that coats the inner surfaces of the eyelids and the outer surface of the eyes.

Disposable product – Intended to be used once for a specific patient, and then discarded.

Durable medical good – Intended for long-term use, though they are to be cleaned between each use.

Infusion – The controlled flow of an intravenous medication into a patient.

Intermittent infusions – Small-volume parenterals.

Intravenous – Injected into the veins.

Parenteral – Bypassing the skin and gastrointestinal tract; injected.

Piggyback – A second intravenous solution, usually of smaller volume than a primary IV, which is administered using a Y-site (or different type) of connection on the primary IV tubing; also known as a *rider*, and is abbreviated as "IVPB" (meaning "intravenous piggyback").

Reusable product – Intended for limited use, with cleaning taking place between each use.

Total parenteral nutrition (TPN) – Nutrition system involving the intravenous infusion of lipids, proteins, electrolytes, sugars, salts, vitamins, and essential elements directly into a vein.

OVERVIEW

Parenteral products are injected directly into body tissue through the skin and veins. Therefore, parenteral administration bypasses the skin and gastrointestinal tract, which are the body's natural barriers to infection. Parenteral products must be produced in a sterile environment to reduce the risk of infection that administration of these products imposes. Sterile preparations must be kept pure and free from biological, chemical, and physical contaminants. The pharmaceutical industry strives to maintain good manufacturing practices of parenteral dosage forms as a result. Likewise, pharmacists and technicians must practice good aseptic technique when working with these products.

PARENTERAL PREPARATIONS

Parenteral preparations are given when a medication is rendered inactive in the gastrointestinal tract or when a patient is unable to take medication by mouth (due to vomiting or unconsciousness). Fluids, electrolytes, and nutrients are often administered parenterally.

Parenteral products must have the following unique qualities:

- They must be sterile.

- They must be free from contamination by endotoxins.

- They must be free from visible particles, which includes reconstitute[d] sterile powders.

- They should be isotonic; the correct level of isotonicity depends o[n] the route of administration.

- They must be chemically, physically, and microbiologically stable.

- They must be compatible with IV delivery systems, diluents, an[d] other drug products to be co-administered.

For administration, injections may be classified in these si[x] categories:

- Solutions ready for injection.

- Dry and soluble products ready for combination with a solvent jus[t] prior to use.

- Suspensions ready for injection.

- Dry, insoluble products ready for combination with a vehicle jus[t] prior to use.

- Emulsions.

- Liquid concentrates ready to be diluted prior to administration.

Formulation modifications, or different routes of injection, ca[n] be used to slow a drug's onset, and thus prolong its action. Parentera[l] administration more readily controls the therapeutic response of a dru[g] because intestinal absorption is bypassed. Disadvantages of parentera[l] administration, however, include the following:

- Asepsis required at administration.

- Risk of tissue toxicity from local irritation.

- Pain.

- Difficulty in correcting errors.

NON-INJECTABLE PRODUCTS

There are certain non-injectable products that must be sterile for use. These include irrigations and ophthalmic products.

Irrigations

The most common sterile irrigations include gentamicin irrigation solution and surgical antibiotic solution (SAS). These agents, which include sterile water (saline), are used during surgery to irrigate open surgical sites. While not truly aseptic in nature, they must be compounded in a sterile environment using sterile IV bottles or bags. The labels of these types of irrigations state that they are to be used *for irrigation only*, and they are never to be used intravenously.

Ophthalmics

Ophthalmics are sterile preparations intended for direct administration into the **conjunctiva** of the eye. Ophthalmic drops contain filtered elements that are safe to use. Ophthalmics are compounded in laminar-airflow hoods in aseptic conditions, then autoclaved for sterilization. They are then cultured to assure that they contain no contaminants. The process for compounding ophthalmics properly takes from 1 to 2 weeks.

INTRAVENOUS PRODUCTS

Intravenous products are injected into the veins. They must be completely sterile. Intravenous products may be small-volume parenterals (SVPs) or large-volume parenterals (LVPs).

Small-Volume Parenteral

Small-volume parenterals (SVPs) are usually 100 mL or less and are primarily used as vehicles for delivering medications. They are generally contained in ampules, vials, prefilled syringes, or in **piggyback** (a second intravenous solution, usually of smaller volume than a primary IV) IVs (Figure 9-1). Medications given with piggybacks usually contain 50 to 100 mL and are typically infused over a period of 30 to 60 minutes.

A piggyback **infusion** is also known as a *rider*, and is abbreviated as "IVPB". Antibiotics given intravenously are routinely piggybacked. Giving antibiotics in this manner, with additional fluids being infused simultaneously, dilutes them further so that they are less irritating to the veins.

Large-Volume Parenteral

Large-volume parenterals (LVPs) are different from small-volume infusions because they can deliver large quantities of fluids, electrolytes, total parenteral nutrition solutions, or chemotherapy. Popular large-volume parenterals include 0.9% sodium chloride, 5% dextrose in water (D_5W), lactated Ringer's, 5% dextrose, and 0.9% sodium chloride (Figure 9-2). Other premixed solutions may contain magnesium, lidocaine, aminophylline,

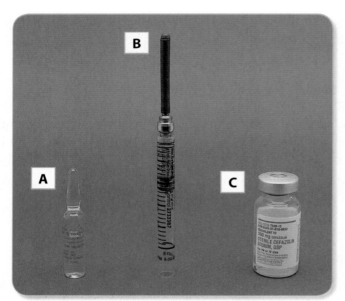

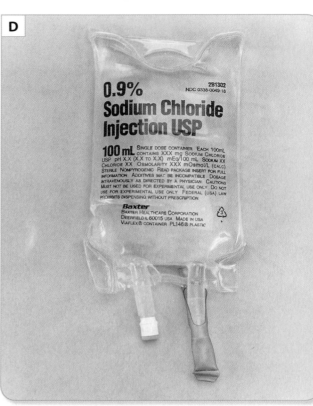

Figure 9-1 Small-volume parenterals (A) Ampule, (B) Prefilled syringe, (C) Vial, (D) Piggyback minibag. (Courtesy of Baxter Healthcare Corporation.)

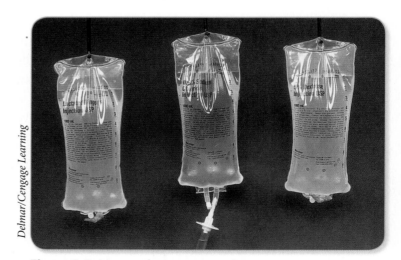

Delmar/Cengage Learning

Figure 9-2 Large-volume parenterals.

nitroglycerin, dopamine, and potassium. When large-volume parenterals require compounding in the pharmacy, it is important that the pharmacist ensures the stability, compatibility, and safety of the mixture. The pharmacist should also verify any high doses of drugs or electrolytes with the physician who orders the compounded large-volume parenteral.

Total Parenteral Nutrition

Total parenteral nutrition (TPN) provides lipids, proteins, electrolytes, sugars, salts, vitamins, and essential elements designed to meet the entire nutritional needs of the patient. It is indicated for patients with severe gastrointestinal (GI) distress, those with poor nutrient absorption, and those who cannot eat. This system of nutrition may be used for patients who have AIDS, cancer, Crohn's disease, severe diarrhea, hyperemesis gravidarum, or surgical removal of the intestines. Premature neonates and comatose patients may also receive total parenteral nutrition. This method of nutrition is infused directly into a vein, usually over a 10- to 12-hour period.

Careful compounding procedures must be followed when working with total parenteral nutrition solutions. Levels of added ingredients must be carefully balanced to ensure that no harm will come to the patient. After the pharmacist or pharmacy technician has made the pertinent mixture calculations, they must be double-checked by a pharmacist.

FACTORS AFFECTING PARENTERAL PRODUCTS

These factors control the choice of a parenteral product's formulation and dosage form:

- Rute of administration – Intravenous, subcutaneous, intradermal, intramuscular, intra-articular, and intrathecal; the type of dosage form will determine the route of administration, and the route of administration will place requirements on the formulation.

- Pharmacokinetics – Rates of absorption for any routes of administration besides intravenous or intra-arterial, rates of distribution, rates of metabolism, and rates of excretion will have an effect on the selected route of administration and type of formulation.

- Solubility – Solubility dictates the concentration of a drug in its dosage form; if the drug is insufficiently soluble in water at the required dosage, the formulation must contain a co-solvent or a solute that increases and maintains the drug in the solution.

- Stability – Stability is sometimes affected by drug concentration; if the drug has significant degradation problems in solution, then a freeze-dried or other sterile solid dosage form must be developed.

- Compatibility – A drug must be compatible with potential formulation additives; this requires pre-formulation screening studies to assure that additives will not cause additional problems with the preparation.

- Packaging – The desired type of packaging is often based on marketing preferences and competition; formulation scientists should know the intended type of packaging early in the developmental process so that the correct formulation may be accomplished.

ADMINISTRATION TECHNIQUES

The mode of IV drug administration depends on the drug used, the patient's condition, and the desired effects of the drug. Generally, the mode of IV drug administration is specified by the physician or another qualified provider. Intravenous medications that are given parenterally may be administered via intermittent or continuous infusion or by rapid direct injection (IV push or bolus).

Intermittent Infusion

In an **intermittent infusion**, a drug is added to between 25 mL and 250 mL of fluid, and then infused over 15 to 90 minutes at specific intervals. In this method, a drug may periodically produce peak blood concentrations. This decreases potential fluid overload, which is better for the patient. Intermittent infusion is usually used for administering IV antibiotics. The four common methods of intermittent infusion are as follows:

- Piggyback infusion – through the pathway of a primary IV.
- Simultaneous infusion – by attaching a second drug to a lower secondary IV port.
- Volume control set – a drug is added to a small amount of solution and infused at a desired rate.
- Direct venous access – a venous access device (for example, a peripheral saline lock or a centrally placed catheter used long term)

Continuous Infusion

This method involves the continuous infusion (over several hours or days) of a drug admixture in a large amount of solution. Using a venous access device for infusion, the container of solution is connected to an administration set. This method is used when constant plasma drug concentration is required, for highly diluted drugs, and when large amounts of electrolytes and fluid must be replaced in the body. Continuous infusion is commonly used for the administration of nitroprusside or potassium chloride.

Rapid Direct Injection

Also known as "bolus" or "IV push," rapid direct injection helps to achieve high serum concentrations of a drug. It involves direct drug administration into a venous access device or through a continuous infusion set's proximal injection port. There may be a greater risk of adverse effects when rapid direct injection is used. Often, this type of injection requires that a prefilled syringe must be used or the drug must be drawn into a syringe before it can be administered. Short needles (usually less than 1 inch long) are used for rapid direct injection to avoid puncturing the vascular access device or the IV tubing.

INTRAVENOUS THERAPY EQUIPMENT

Intravenous therapy equipment is divided into three groups: disposable products, durable medical goods, and reusable products. **Disposable products** are intended to be used once for a specific patient and then discarded. Many intravenous products, including administration sets, catheters, containers, and dressings, are disposable. **Durable medical goods** are intended for long-term use, though they are to be cleaned between each use. Durable goods include infusion pumps, IV poles, walkers, and wheelchairs. **Reusable products** are intended for limited use, with cleaning taking place between each use. These items, which must be designated "reusable," include certain types of needles and syringes, instrument organizers, certain types of drapes, and certain ice packs.

An infusion device is one that regulates the infusion of an intravenous substance, controlling the flow of medication into a patient. Infusion pumps are important in the home health care setting to ensure accurate infusion at all times. The choice of an infusion device relates to the choice of an IV container such as a bag, syringe, or elastomeric balloon (a pressurized balloon reservoir from which medication is infused by the deflation of the balloon).

Stationary infusion pumps attach to IV poles and are used for patients who are confined to their beds or who need infusion therapy during the night. Ambulatory infusion pumps are small and portable, and can be worn by patients who are not confined to bed.

Pharmacy technicians must protect patients from any harm that may be caused by the incorrect use of medical goods and products. Proper training of personnel is essential so that all goods, products, and equipment are used correctly. All equipment must be in good repair, free from potential hazards, and used only for the purposes specified by the manufacturer.

Infusion equipment must be inspected for quality three times—before, during, and after use. No potentially harmful piece of infusion equipment should ever be used. All products or equipment of this type that may be potentially harmful should be reported according to the workplace's established guidelines.

PREPARATION OF PARENTERAL PRODUCTS

Parenteral products must be prepared with strict controls to avoid contamination. Parenteral products can be contaminated by contact with health care personnel, supply air, particle infiltration, and contaminants on equipment. Giving a patient a contaminated product can cause serious adverse effects, including death. Parenteral medications account for more than 40 percent of all medications administered in institutional practice.

Laminar-Airflow Hoods

Aseptic technique (preparing and handling sterile products in a manner that prevents microbial contamination) must be strictly applied when preparing parenteral products. The work area must be tightly controlled to assure cleanliness in order to prevent contamination from any source. Clean areas may be easily provided by the use of laminar-airflow hoods, used in conjunction with proper aseptic technique.

Laminar-airflow hoods filter air through high-efficiency particulate air (HEPA) filters that flow through the hood in straight and parallel lines and remove 99.97 percent of all particles larger than 0.3 μm in size (all microbial contaminants and particulate matter). Laminar-airflow moves fast enough to keep the work area from becoming contaminated, in either a horizontal or a vertical direction. See Chapter 7 for more in-depth information about laminar-airflow hoods and aseptic technique.

Role of the Technician

The role of the pharmacy technician in handling sterile preparations and the procedures of compounding are varied. These activities include:

- In-depth knowledge of sterile compounding.
- Excellent aseptic technique.
- Skill and knowledge of pharmaceutical calculations.
- Familiarity with parenteral devices and equipment.
- Labeling of sterile products.
- Completing of compounding records.
- Performing quality control activities in the compounding area.
- Cleaning and disinfection the compounding area.
- Completing cleaning logs.
- Ordering, receiving, and stocking IV medications and compounding supplies.
- Picking, assembling, and packaging of the appropriate equipment and supplies, and arranging for their delivery.
- Excellent computer skills.
- Knowledge of the legislation and regulations pertaining to sterile compounding.

Alert

The pharmacy technician involved in sterile compounding works under the direct supervision of a pharmacist.

United States Pharmacopoeia (USP) Chapter <797>

Chapter <797> of the United States Pharmacopoeia was published in 2004, and set standards for the compounding, preparing, and labeling of sterile drug preparations. It has provisions for home infusion pharmacies that are required and enforced by the FDA and the state boards of pharmacy. The most important issues applying to home infusion pharmacies are beyond-use dating and the maintenance of quality sterile drug preparations once they leave the pharmacy.

According to USP, the **beyond-use date** is calculated from the time that a sterile drug product is compounded until it is administered to a patient. There are three risk levels for contamination of sterile products under the USP, high, medium, and low, as follows:

Risk	Time at Room Temp	Refrigerate for
High	24 hours	3 days
Medium	30 hours	7 days
Low	48 hours	14 days

Drugs of all risk levels can be frozen for up to 45 days. Compounded sterile products should not be shaken, exposed to excessive light, or exposed to excessive heat. Both the patient and caregiver should be trained about the proper storage of sterile drug products in the home.

Exercise

Objective: To become familiar with the beyond-use date of a specific product, as specified by the USP.

Select a sterile drug product, compounded according to the USP, and calculate the beyond-use date (at medium risk level) for contamination of the sterile product.

Compounding Records

A compounding record is also known as a *mixing report*. It may be a computerized or paper record. Compounding records are used to document the activities that are undertaken during compounding. They are stored along with patient charts. A compounding record includes the following information: expiration dates of the substances used, lot numbers, stability information about the final mixture, and specific compounding instructions for the mixture (Figure 9-3).

Exercise

Objective: To become familiar with the information required on a compounding record.

Complete all information on a compounding record by using a computer and printing out the results.

MIXING REPORT

Stability:	Patient Name:
Reference: *Handbook of Inj. Drugs*	Origin Rx Number:
Other:	
Calculations: Checked By	Place copy of Rx label here:

Refill Date	Ingredients (one per line)	Volume used	Units used	Prepared date–time	MFG lot no.	Exp. date	Prep. by:

Figure 9-3 Compounding report.

Policies and Procedures for Sterile Product Preparation

Before compounding sterile products, health care personnel should read their facility's policies and procedures, and verify by signature that they have done so. The following topics should be covered by the policies and procedures manual concerning sterile product preparation:

- Job description – education level; certification; registration; length of experience; type of experience; ability to lift various weights; ability to push carts; ability to do rapid, repetitive, and accurate manipulations; work shifts; environment; garb; ability to compound pharmaceutical products that are free of contaminants.

- Job orientation – roles of employees; garb; facilities; equipment; area-specific techniques; reference materials.

- Training and education – aseptic technique and quality control; chemical, pharmaceutical, and clinical properties of drugs; good manufacturing practices; equipment operation; product handling.

- Competency evaluation – methods of observation and/or testing; intervals between evaluations; aseptic technique; handling new equipment; written math skills tests.

- Acquisition – ingredient selection; bulk drug substance dating procedures; repackaging guidelines; identification of ingredients by testing; purchasing equipment, containers, and closure.

- Storage – temperature monitoring of refrigerators and freezers, light, ventilation, and humidity; stock rotation and inspection; locations of quarantined products.

- Handling – removal of outer packaging in anterooms; handling of pouched supplies; decontamination of ampules and vials; disposal of used items, hazardous wastes, and sharps; inspection of sterile ingredients and containers prior to compounding; handling expired drugs and supplies; handling product recalls.

- Facilities – cleaning procedures; traffic control; safety.

- Equipment – location; use; cleaning; cart entry past demarcation line in the anteroom; laminar-airflow hoods; traffic.

- Personal conduct and garb – eating; drinking; smoking; wearing makeup and jewelry; hand washing and drying; dealing with infectious conditions; garb policies and procedures.

- Other important areas – product integrity, aseptic technique, work sheets, batch preparation records, sterilization methods, environmental monitoring, process validation, expiration dating, labeling, end-product valuation, maintaining quality of compounded products, patient monitoring, housekeeping, quality assurance, and documentation records.

PROCEDURES FOR HANDLING AND PREPARING PARENTERAL PRODUCTS

Pharmacy technicians must follow the policies and procedures of the pharmacy concerning sterile compounding. The goal is to handle and prepare parenteral preparations in a manner that is as free from biological, chemical, and physical contaminants as possible. This requires proper aseptic technique because parenteral preparations are often unstable and highly potent—their characteristics must be preserved without contaminating them. Important properties of parenteral preparations that must be considered include compatibility, osmolality (concentration of particles or substances), osmolarity (concentration of diffused, active particles), pH, stability, and tonicity (tone or tension of a substance).

Visual Inspection of the Parenteral Product

It is important to visually inspect parenteral products to check for cloudiness, color changes, or other conditions that can demonstrate the product may be contaminated, defective, or otherwise unusable. The policies and procedures manual of the sterile compounding facility requires that parenteral products be visually inspected. A parenteral product that is contaminated or defective may cause harm to the patient.

Alert

Parenteral solutions must always be visually inspected before use.

Procedure: *Visually Inspecting a Parenteral Solution before Use*

Objective: To properly determine that a parenteral solution is in acceptable condition to use and is not contaminated or damaged in any way.

Equipment Needed: parenteral product

Step 1: Inspect the parenteral solution container for any damage and proper seal.

Step 2: Read the label.

Step 3: Verify that it is the correct medication required for use (Figure 9-4A).

Step 4: Verify that it is not expired.

Step 5: Turn the container upside down. Using good lighting, inspect the container for any clouding, hazing, or particles in the solution (Figure 9-4B).

Step 6: If there is no visible contamination and the container is properly sealed, it may be used.

Step 7: If there is any visible contamination or the container is not properly sealed, it should be discarded properly.

Procedure: (Continued)

Figure 9-4 Visual inspection of a parenteral product. (A) Read the label and verify that it is the correct medication. (B) Turn the container upside down look for hazing, cloudiness, and particulates in the solution.

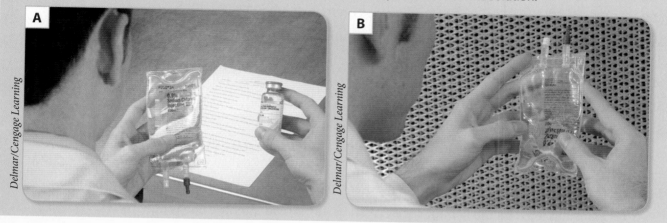

Exercise

Objective: To become familiar with the proper inspection techniques for an IV bag.

Practice visually inspecting a sample parenteral solution for proper quality.

Preparation of IV Admixtures

Intravenous admixtures consist of several sterile products added into an IV fluid for administration. They must be mixed using aseptic technique. This may be accomplished by mixing them inside a laminar-airflow hood. Each sterile product should be added into the IV fluid with a fresh disposable syringe. Some IV admixtures, such as antibiotics, may be frozen after mixing due to the limited stability they may have after being mixed—as long as they are not intended for immediate use. Others do not have to be frozen, but must be used within a short period of time after being mixed.

Procedure: Adding a Medication to an IV Bag

Objective: To demonstrate the proper technique used to add a medication to an existing IV bag.

Equipment Needed: primary IV, drug additive, alcohol swab, needle and syringe, label

Step 1: Review the medication order.

Step 2: Check for any drug allergies.

Procedure: (Continued)

Step 3: Make sure that the drug to be added to the IV bag is compatible with the existing IV solution.

Step 4: Wash your hands.

Step 5: Clean the IV bag's injection port with an alcohol swab.

Step 6: Insert the needle of the syringe containing the drug to be added into the IV bag's injection port (Figure 9-5A).

Step 7: Inject the drug into the bag.

Step 8: Withdraw the needle from the port.

Step 9: Rotate the IV bag gently (this will mix the solution).

Step 10: Inspect the solution for any separation of the ingredients (you can only use the mixed solution if there is no separation) (Figure 9-5B).

Step 11: Note the date, time, drug name, and dosage of the additive on the medication label.

Step 12: Place this label on the IV bag so that it can be easily read after the bag is hung.

Step 13: The mixed solution is now ready to be administered to the patient.

Figure 9-5 Preparing an IV admixture. (A) Insert the syringe into the port on the IV bag (B) Check the medication in the bag.

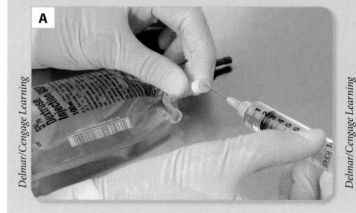
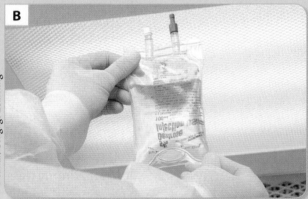

Delmar/Cengage Learning

Procedure: Parenteral Compounding

Objective: To demonstrate the proper procedure for compounding a parenteral while maintaining the integrity of the product.

Equipment Needed: laminar-airflow hood, PPE, alcohol, materials to be compounded, filters, needles, syringes, parenteral container

Step 1: Cycle the flow hood for at least 30 minutes before using.

Step 2: Wear protective clothing.

Step 3: Clean the flow hood with 70% isopropyl alcohol (or other approved disinfectant), moving from back to front, then cleaning the bottom of the hood.

Procedure: *(Continued)*

Step 4: Collect the substances that must be compounded.

Step 5: Check expiration dates of all substances (Figure 9-6A).

Step 6: Check for any leaks in bags.

Step 7: Remove any dust coverings.

Step 8: Only use pre-sterilized filters, needles, and syringes.

Step 9: Position supplies in the hood (Figure 9-6B).

Step 10: Sterilize puncture surfaces with alcohol wipes.

Step 11: Draw a volume of air into the syringe that is equal to the volume being replaced (Figure 9-6C).

Step 12: Puncture vial with proper 45- to 60-degree angles using downward pressure while vial is placed on a flat surface; move needle to a 90-degree angle (Figures 9–6D and E).

Step 13: Invert the vial and pull back on the plunger to fill the syringe, tapping it so that any air bubbles come to the top (Figure 9-6F).

Step 14: Transfer the solution into the final container (Figure 9-6G).

Figure 9-6 Compounding a parenteral product. (A) Check the expiration dates on all products to be combined (B) Position the supplies in the laminar-airflow hood (C) Draw air into the syringe (D) Insert the syringe at a 45-degree angle.

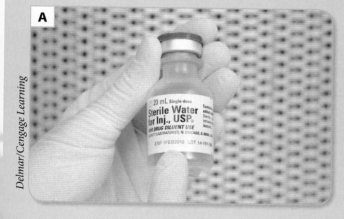

Delmar/Cengage Learning

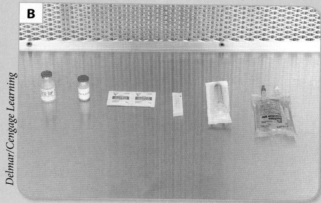

Delmar/Cengage Learning

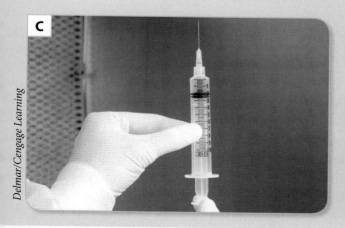

Delmar/Cengage Learning

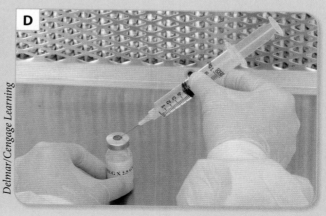

Delmar/Cengage Learning

Procedure: (Continued)

Figure 9-6 Compounding a parenteral product. (E) Move the syringe to a 90-degree angle (F) Invert vial and fill syringe with medication (G) Instill medication into final container.

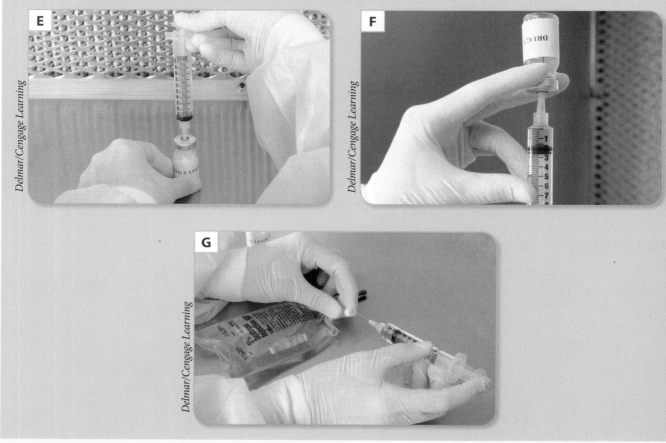

Compounding a TPN Product

TPN solutions are compounded in laminar-airflow hoods or in biologica safety cabinets (BSCs). The base solution is composed of dextrose, amino acids, sterile water for injection, and sometimes lipids. Additives that are mixed into the base solution may include electrolytes, minerals, vitamins and other prescribed substances. TPN solutions may be compounded either by hand or by using automated mixing devices.

When choosing a bag to contain the TPN solution, the bag that i the smallest size in which the entire finished mixed solution will fit shoul be chosen. The base components must be mixed in the following order t ensure proper formulation: dextrose, amino acids, lipids, and sterile wate for injection (SWFI). The additives are then injected separately into the TPN bag after the pharmacist performs a final check as to their accuracy. The bag should be gently mixed after the addition of each additive. Lipids shoul always be added last because they can mask particulates or precipitation in the final solution. After all additives have been injected, gently rotate or shake the bag to blend all the ingredients evenly.

A standard total parenteral solution is as follows: 42.5 g of amino acid and 250 g of dextrose (500 mL of an 8.5% amino acid solution and 500 mL of 50% dextrose) per liter. This formula provides 1,000 calories per liter, with a non-protein-calorie-to-nitrogen ratio of 150:1. To prevent essential fatty acid deficiency, IV lipids are usually provided separately twice per week. Before administering the TPN solution, verify with the facility's procedures whether any inline filters should be used.

There are automated filling devices that may be used to compound total parenteral solutions. These are linked to computers to help control accuracy. When a pharmacist or pharmacy technician receives an order for a total parenteral solution, he or she should enter the information from the prescription into the automated filling device's computer to calculate the amounts of each ingredient. The computer has automatic warning software that will alert the operator to any possible problems. Labels will be generated for the solution to be compounded, and these should be checked and re-checked. The compounding device should be programmed for the correct patient, and the TPN bag hung appropriately so that it can be filled. The device weighs the filled bag to ascertain accuracy. Each ingredient is pumped into the TPN bag in a specific sequence. The device can detect if the specific gravity is incorrect for any of the ingredients, and will alert the operator if this occurs. Newer types of automated filling devices can handle more complex mixtures of TPN ingredients.

Preparing an IV Piggyback

IV piggybacks may be prepared in several ways depending on the type of equipment used. In the traditional method, a vial of medication is added to an IV medication by removing the contents of the vial via a syringe and injecting it into the IV bag of medication. A newer method allows a vial to be attached to an IV bag without actually mixing the contents beforehand. In this method, the medications are mixed at the time they are administered, and not before. This method usually allows for longer expiration dates than in the traditional method. If antibiotics are activated in an IV piggyback, these products must be refrigerated, and should be labeled accordingly.

SUMMARY

Non-injectable products include irrigations (used for open surgical sites) and ophthalmics (intended for direct administration into the conjunctiva of the eye). Parenteral products include intravenous products (either small-volume or large-volume parenterals) and total parenteral nutrition. Small-volume parenterals consist of secondary or "piggyback" IVs, which are added to large-volume parenterals (also known as primary IVs). A parenteral product may be chosen based upon its route of administration, pharmacokinetics, solubility, stability, compatibility, and packaging. Total parenteral nutrition (TPN) is designed to meet the entire nutritional needs of patients who cannot eat, cannot absorb nutrients properly, or have severe gastrointestinal distress. Parenteral products are commonly administered by IV push, infusion, or intravenous piggyback (IVPB).

Parenteral products must be prepared with strict control to avoid contamination, commonly in laminar-airflow hoods. Standards for the correct procedures of compounding, preparing, and labeling of sterile drug preparations are set forth in the United States Pharmacopoeia (USP) Chapter <797>. This includes beyond-use dates, which are calculated from the time a sterile drug product is compounded until it is administered to a patient.

REVIEW QUESTIONS

Multiple Choice

1. The most important characteristic of an injectable solution is:

   A. viscosity
   B. dispensability

   C. sterility
   D. color

2. Which of the following are most commonly used for the compounding of IV antibiotics?

   A. intravenous piggybacks
   B. large-volume bags

   C. irrigations
   D. syringes

3. Which of the following is the base solution for compounding total parenteral nutrition?

   A. sterile water
   B. amino acid

   C. dextrose
   D. all of the above

4. According to the USP, high-risk compounding products can be kept in a refrigerator for:

   A. 6 hours
   B. 24 hours

   C. 48 hours
   D. 72 hours

5. Which of the following base components must be mixed last into a TPN bag?

   A. dextrose
   B. lipids
   C. sterile water
   D. amino acids

6. Large-volume parenterals can deliver large quantities of all of the following, except:

   A. chemotherapy
   B. antibiotics
   C. electrolytes
   D. total parenteral nutrition solutions

7. Ophthalmics are compounded in laminar-airflow hoods for which of the following purposes?

   A. sterilization
   B. destruction of spores
   C. aseptic conditions
   D. all of the above

8. Sterile irrigations are used for:

   A. intravenous injections
   B. rehydration
   C. surgical sites
   D. all of the above

9. Medications given via the parenteral route may be administered via which of the following?

   A. rapid direct injection
   B. continuous infusion
   C. intermittent infusion
   D. all of the above

10. Parenteral products must be prepared with strict controls to avoid:

   A. expiration
   B. contamination
   C. lysation
   D. none of the above

Fill in the Blank

1. Vials may be single-use or _____.

2. Clean areas may be easily provided and regulated by the use of _____.

3. Chapter <797> of the United States Pharmacopoeia was published in _____.

4. There are _____ risk levels for contamination of sterile products under the USP.

5. In the IV push system, a medication is contained in a _____.

6. The choice of an infusion device relates to the choice of an IV _____ such as a bag, syringe, or elastomeric balloon.

7. The process for compounding ophthalmics properly takes _____ weeks.

8. A piggyback is a _____ intravenous solution, usually of smaller volume than a primary IV.

9. Lipids are added last to TPN solutions because they can mask particulates or _____ in the final solution.

10. Parenteral medications account for more than _____ percent of all medications administered in institutional practice.

Inventory Control

OBJECTIVES

Upon completion of this chapter, the student should be able to:

1. Identify the pharmacy technician's inventory control responsibilities.
2. Explain the stocking of shelves in the hospital pharmacy.
3. Define the terms "shelf life" and "expiration date".
4. Describe how to keep track of inventory and the "eyeball inventory" system.
5. Explain the procedures for ordering and receiving pharmaceutical products.
6. Explain the importance of controlled substance inventory.
7. Identify drug storage requirements.
8. Explain the stocking of shelves in the home infusion pharmacy.

GLOSSARY

Back-ordered – Temporarily unavailable from the supplier; also known as *short*.

Chart orders – A prescriber's instructions for diet, nursing care, laboratory tests, medications, and treatments for an inpatient.

Expiration date – A date, assigned by a drug's manufacturer, after which its stability and potency can no longer be guaranteed; also known as its *beyond-use date*.

Invoice – Bill for goods received.

NDC number – A unique number identifying a drug product; it indicates the manufacturer's name, drug strength, dosage form, and package size.

Perpetual inventory – Ongoing system of tracking of drugs received by and sold in the pharmacy.

Pharmacy patient profile – A confidential record that contains medical and billing information, along with a list of medications received by the patient.

Shelf life – The length of time a drug remains potent.

OVERVIEW

A pharmacy's goal is to provide the best patient service possible while minimizing operating costs. The drug inventory in a pharmaceutical compounding pharmacy is generally the same as in other types of pharmacies. However, compounded products have reduced shelf life. Therefore, pharmacy technicians play an important role in the reduction of costs. Maintaining, managing, and accounting for inventory is one of the most important responsibilities of the pharmacy technician. Keeping adequate amounts of medications and supplies is critical to maintaining good patient service. Pharmacy technicians will find that a large portion of their job requirements in the compounding pharmacy includes stocking shelves and ordering supplies. The importance of these duties cannot be overstated.

Inventory control involves maintaining an adequate stock of medications, as well as storing medications in a safe and secure manner. It also means keeping track of the purchasing and distribution of medications. Good inventory control allows the pharmacy to have enough medication on hand to fill prescriptions and orders for compounding, without having so much stock that drugs deteriorate before they can be used.

ROLE OF THE TECHNICIAN IN INVENTORY

The responsibilities of pharmacy technicians in inventory control include:

- Following the policies and procedures of inventory control.
- Providing accurate inventory records.
- Determining sources of pharmaceutical products.
- Identifying and ordering needed pharmaceutical products.
- Receiving and storing pharmaceutical products.
- Removing obsolete or expired products.

Exercise

Objective: To get in the habit of checking expiration dates and become familiar with proper disposal of expired drugs.

Check the drug shelves and remove all obsolete or expired products in the pharmacy laboratory.

SHELF LIFE

A drug's **shelf life** is based on its stability and describes the length of time it can be kept in stock before its contents become altered. Each manufacturer indicates the shelf life of the drugs they market by assigning an **expiration date** or a *beyond-use date*. When a drug has expired, its potency can no longer be guaranteed, so medications should never be sold once they reach their expiration date. Both prescription medications and OTC products must be routinely checked for reaching their expiration dates. Once expired, they must be removed from stock and properly disposed of.

Patients must be instructed never to use their medications past the expiration dates. Though most medications become less effective over time, some actually increase in toxicity and can potentially harm anyone who takes them. Some drugs can lose potency before their expiration date and must be protected by storing in refrigerators and freezers to protect them from excess light and humidity. Pharmacy technicians must ensure that proper storage techniques are followed for each drug that is stocked in the pharmacy.

Exercise

Objective: To become familiar with reading drug labels and storage requirements.

Look at the following labels and review the storage requirements related to temperature, light exposure, and humidity. Please note the specific requirements for each label.

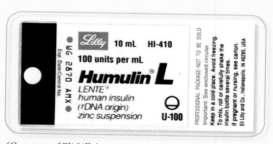

(Courtesy of Eli Lilly)

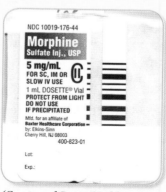

(Courtesy of Baxter Healthcare Corporation)

Exercise (Continued)

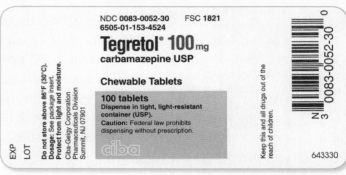

(Courtesy of Novartis Pharmaceutical Corporation)

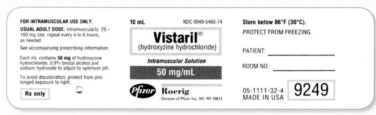

(Courtesy of Pfizer, Inc.)

NDC 10019-940-17

Methotrexate
Injection, USP

PRESERVATIVE FREE Rx only
50 mg (25 mg/mL)
Sterile Isotonic Liquid
2 mL Single Dose Vial

Mfd. for Baxter Healthcare Corp. affiliate
by: Bigmar Pharmaceuticals SA
Barbengo, Switzerland

See package insert for routes of administration.
Usual Dosage: Consult package insert for dosage and full prescribing information.
Each mL contains methotrexate sodium equivalent to 25 mg methotrexate.
Inactive ingredients: Sodium Chloride 0.490% w/v and Water for Injection. Sodium hydroxide and/or hydrochloric acid may be added to adjust pH to 8.5-8.7 during manufacture.
Store at controlled room temperature 15°-30°C (59°-86°F). PROTECT FROM LIGHT. Retain in carton until time of use. Discard any unused portion.   10-1038A   460-222-00

(Courtesy of Baxter Healthcare Corporation)

Humulin L® _____

Morphine _____

Tegretol _____

Vistaril® _____

Methotrexate _____

PURCHASING

Alert!

Before ordering products from manufacturers, the pharmacy must determine if it is cost-effective to order the required quantity of an item in order to get the lower price.

Pharmacies may purchase pharmaceutical products from five differe[nt] sources: manufacturers, wholesalers, purchasing groups, prime vendors, a[nd] other pharmacies. A direct purchase is one that is made directly from th[e] manufacturer by the pharmacy. The manufacturer offers the lowest price a[nd] requires a minimum quantity order. Most prescription drug products a[re] purchased through wholesalers that carry expensive prescription produc[ts] from different manufacturers. Wholesalers also carry over-the-count[er] drugs and other medical supplies, and small items (*sundries*) that inclu[de] bandages, safety pins, sunglasses, etc.

Many medications are purchased by the pharmacy from a "prime vendor," which guarantees a lower price. These agreements may entitle the pharmacy to special services from the vendor. When a medication is **back-ordered** (or "short") from a prime vendor, secondary vendors will be used to avoid unnecessary delays that can cause problems for a patient. Computerized ordering systems use bar codes or numeric identifiers to reduce the chance of ordering an incorrect product. While some vendors use a unique number for each product they carry, others use the manufacturer's National Drug Code (NDC) number. An **NDC number** uniquely identifies each drug product and indicates the manufacturer's name, the drug's name, its strength, its dosage form, and the package size of the drug product.

Inventory should be tracked using either an organized inventory system or an "eyeball inventory" system. On a daily basis, the pharmacy's staff can keep track of medications that are sold by listing them in a "want book,"

Exercise

Objective: To become familiar with reading drug labels.

Find the NDC number for each of the following drugs:

Percocet® _____

Bactrim® _____

Propulsid® _____

Biaxin® _____

Klonopin® _____

Claforan® _____

Lidocaine _____

Methotrexate _____

Inderal® _____

Furosemide _____

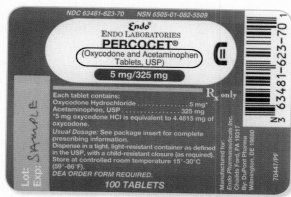

(Courtesy of Endo Pharmaceutical Inc.)

Exercise (Continued)

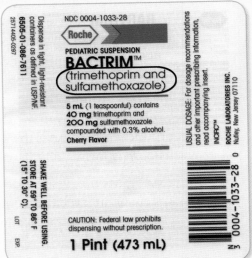

(Courtesy of Roche Laboratories, Inc.)

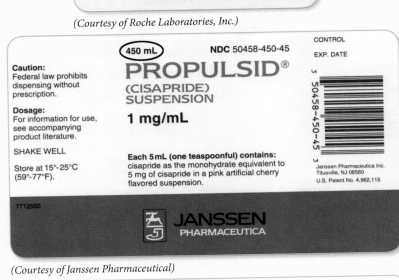

(Courtesy of Janssen Pharmaceutical)

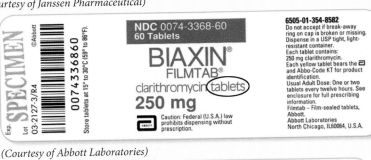

(Courtesy of Abbott Laboratories)

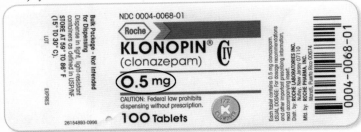

(Courtesy of Roche Laboratories, Inc.)

Exercise (Continued)

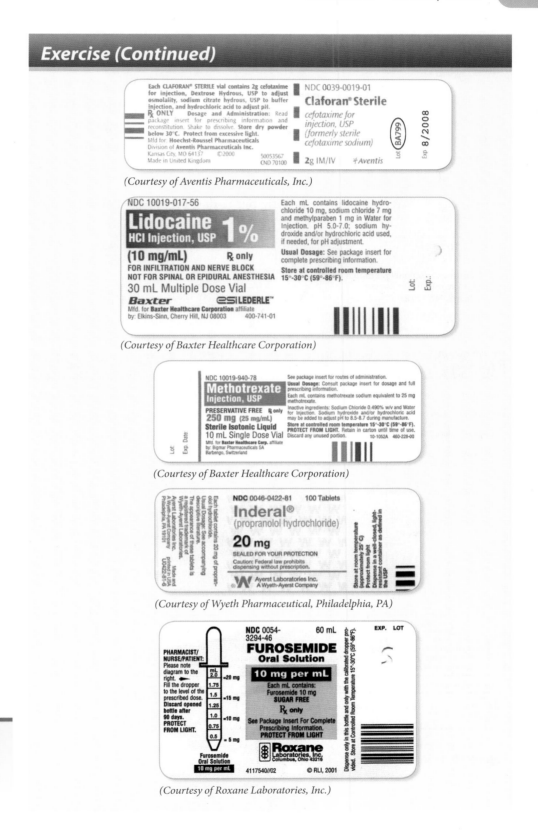

(Courtesy of Aventis Pharmaceuticals, Inc.)

(Courtesy of Baxter Healthcare Corporation)

(Courtesy of Baxter Healthcare Corporation)

(Courtesy of Wyeth Pharmaceutical, Philadelphia, PA)

(Courtesy of Roxane Laboratories, Inc.)

Alert!

A pharmacy may borrow items from another pharmacy if it runs out of an item that it routinely stocks, or is in immediate need of an item that it normally does not stock.

or by entering their numeric identifiers into the computer system. Bar codes have greatly simplified inventory processes as well as sales. These systems keep a **perpetual inventory** of drugs that have been used and automatically create an order for replacement drugs.

RECEIVING SHIPMENTS

Pharmacy technicians must follow the pharmacy's procedures for receiving shipments. The supplier includes an **invoice**, which is a listing of the items in the shipment. The invoice must be checked item by item against the items in the shipment to make sure that nothing is missing, and that there are no items included that were not ordered. After this, you may document the receipt of goods by entering the information into a computer, or by scanning bar codes. Figure 10-1 shows an original invoice with a barcode.

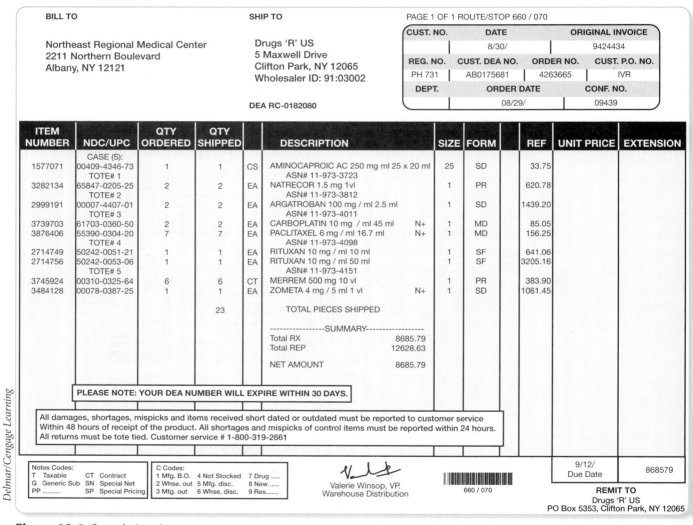

BILL TO

Northeast Regional Medical Center
2211 Northern Boulevard
Albany, NY 12121

SHIP TO

Drugs 'R' US
5 Maxwell Drive
Clifton Park, NY 12065
Wholesaler ID: 91:03002

DEA RC-0182080

PAGE 1 OF 1 ROUTE/STOP 660 / 070

CUST. NO.	DATE		ORIGINAL INVOICE
	8/30/		9424434
REG. NO.	CUST. DEA NO.	ORDER NO.	CUST. P.O. NO.
PH 731	AB0175681	4263665	IVR
DEPT.	ORDER DATE		CONF. NO.
	08/29/		09439

ITEM NUMBER	NDC/UPC	QTY ORDERED	QTY SHIPPED		DESCRIPTION		SIZE	FORM	REF	UNIT PRICE	EXTENSION
	CASE (S):										
1577071	00409-4346-73	1	1	CS	AMINOCAPROIC AC 250 mg ml 25 x 20 ml		25	SD	33.75		
	TOTE# 1				ASN# 11-973-3723						
3282134	65847-0205-25	2	2	EA	NATRECOR 1.5 mg 1vl		1	PR	620.78		
	TOTE# 2				ASN# 11-973-3812						
2999191	00007-4407-01	2	2	EA	ARGATROBAN 100 mg / ml 2.5 ml		1	SD	1439.20		
	TOTE# 3				ASN# 11-973-4011						
3739703	61703-0360-50	2	2	EA	CARBOPLATIN 10 mg / ml 45 ml	N+	1	MD	85.05		
3876406	55390-0304-20	7	7	EA	PACLITAXEL 6 mg / ml 16.7 ml	N+	1	MD	156.25		
	TOTE# 4				ASN# 11-973-4098						
2714749	50242-0051-21	1	1	EA	RITUXAN 10 mg / ml 10 ml		1	SF	641.06		
2714756	50242-0053-06	1	1	EA	RITUXAN 10 mg / ml 50 ml		1	SF	3205.16		
	TOTE# 5				ASN# 11-973-4151						
3745924	00310-0325-64	6	6	CT	MERREM 500 mg 10 vl		1	PR	383.90		
3484128	00078-0387-25	1	1	EA	ZOMETA 4 mg / 5 ml 1 vl	N+	1	SD	1061.45		
			23		TOTAL PIECES SHIPPED						

-----------------SUMMARY-----------------
Total RX   8685.79
Total REP   12628.63

NET AMOUNT   8685.79

PLEASE NOTE: YOUR DEA NUMBER WILL EXPIRE WITHIN 30 DAYS.

All damages, shortages, mispicks and items received short dated or outdated must be reported to customer service Within 48 hours of receipt of the product. All shortages and mispicks of control items must be reported within 24 hours. All returns must be tote tied. Customer service # 1-800-319-2661

Notes Codes:		C Codes:			
T Taxable	CT Contract	1 Mfg. B.O.	4 Not Stocked	7 Drug	
G Generic Sub	SN Special Net	2 Whse. out	5 Mfg. disc.	8 New	
PP	SP Special Pricing	3 Mtg. out	6 Whse. disc.	9 Res.......	

Valerie Winsop, VP.
Warehouse Distribution

660 / 070

9/12/
Due Date

868579

REMIT TO
Drugs 'R' US
PO Box 5353, Clifton Park, NY 12065

Delmar/Cengage Learning

Figure 10-1 Sample invoice.

Exercise

Objective: To become familiar with the process of receiving drugs into stock.

Select 10 random empty drug containers and list them as if they were all received in a single shipment. Practice entering a receipt of inventory for this shipment into a computer.

RETURNING ITEMS

After checking all items against the orders that you receive, you may find that some items are defective, some products are expired, or the supplier has overshipped certain items. The pharmacy technician must use appropriate return forms when returning goods. On a return form, the following information must be included:

- Original purchase order (p.o.) number.

- Item number.

- Quantity.

- Reason for return (see Figure 10-2).

Please complete the form below if you would like to initiate a request to return goods. Your request will be reviewed by our Customer Service Department. You will receive a Return Goods Authorization Number and shipping instructions after your return request has been approved. A Customer Service Representative will contact you if any additional information is needed.

RETURNED GOODS REQUEST FORM

Hazardous Material: Yes ☐ No ☐ Description:	Date:	Facility/Company:
Customer ID:	Contact Name:	Phone #: / Fax #:
Address:	City/State/Zip:	Email Address:
P.O.#:	Packing List #:	Invoice #:

Reason for Return:

Qty	Item Number	Lot Number	Description	Condition	Disposition	Date

Drugs 'R' Us is committed to your total satisfaction. Please call, fax, or email the above information to obtain an RGA#.

Phone: 888-662-4526   Fax: 888-662-5064   E-Mail: customerservice@drugsrus.com

Delmar/Cengage Learning

Figure 10-2 Sample returned goods request form.

CONTROLLED SUBSTANCES

Controlled substances (particularly Schedule II drugs) require detailed record keeping because they have high abuse potential. The DEA has strict guidelines for ordering, receiving, storing, and destroying controlled substances in Schedule II through IV. The pharmacy must use special DEA forms to manage controlled substance inventory.

When orders of controlled substances arrive, they must be signed for by the pharmacist and not by any pharmacy technician. At least every 2 years, each pharmacy must do a physical count of all controlled substances, counting every tablet and every capsule, and recording the counts in an inventory record.

STOCKING SHELVES

Stocking requires a lot of time and knowledge about the pharmacy's arrangement of its drug supply. Storage of drugs must be handled by following the manufacturer's recommendations for temperature, light exposure, humidity, and other factors. This not only helps to save time, but can potentially save the pharmacy a lot of money due to the expense of many drugs that can be easily damaged or rendered infective by improper storage. For safety, different types of drugs should be stored separately from other types. An example would be the storage of oral drugs apart from topical drugs.

Controlled substances are usually stored in locked areas away from other drug products. Only specific people in the pharmacy should have access to controlled substances. Likewise, chemotherapy drugs are usually kept in their own secured area of the pharmacy due to their toxicity and resulting requirements for extra special care and handling.

Once separated into its group of drugs, every medication should be arranged alphabetically. Pharmacies differ in alphabetical storage—some use the drugs' generic names, while others use the trade names. Whenever you are in doubt about a drug's correct name or anything concerning its location in the pharmacy, ask your pharmacist.

Stocking Shelves in the Hospital Pharmacy

Hospital pharmacies stock many more different medications than retail pharmacies because they deal more frequently with inpatients. OTC drugs in the hospital pharmacy are often used along with bulk prescription drugs but are not sold to hospital customers.

The unit-dose system of dispensing oral medications is used in many hospitals, meaning that each package of medication only contains a single dose. This system reduces cross-contamination and the chance of medication errors. It also decreases pharmacy staff time. While many medications are available pre-packaged in unit-dose containers, some are not. This requires the hospital pharmacy to buy these medications in bulk containers, and repackage them into unit doses.

Many medications for hospital patients are in injectable form because many hospitalized patients are sicker than those treated by retail (outpatient) pharmacies. Intravenous (IV) medications are commonly stored in the hospital pharmacy. IV mixtures are prepared inside laminar-airflow hoods within a clean room within the hospital pharmacy to minimize risk of contamination.

Since many IV medications have short shelf lives, their admixtures are prepared when needed by a patient. This reduces waste, but requires the clean room in a hospital pharmacy to be able to operate 24 hours a day.

DRUG DISTRIBUTION IN THE HOSPITAL PHARMACY

In the hospital, when a prescriber writes a drug order on the patient's chart, pharmacy technicians then collect copies of the charts and begin the process of medication distribution. The symbols and abbreviations used on **chart orders** are the same as those used on prescriptions. Chart orders are often picked up on an hourly basis from nursing stations. Chart orders can also be electronically transmitted to the hospital pharmacy.

In the hospital pharmacy, medication orders are entered in a **pharmacy patient profile** that lists all of the medications a patient is to receive, regardless of frequency of administration. The pharmacy patient profile is updated when new medications are ordered and previous orders are changed or discontinued. Patient diagnoses and medical history may be included on these profiles. This information helps the pharmacist to monitor the patient and response to drug therapy.

Often, the pharmacy patient profile is computerized and available throughout the hospital, in some cases used as part of the nursing staff's Medication Administration Record (MAR). MARs are legal records of all patient doses that have been received. They become part of the patient's chart and are also used for billing records.

Unit-Dose Distribution

In unit-dose distribution, medications for patients are usually distributed in cubicles or cassettes, one per patient, that are labeled with the patient's name, room number, and medical record number. Medication carts used by nurses contain these cassettes, which are fitted into cartridges, locked into the carts for protection from tampering or theft (Figure 10-3).

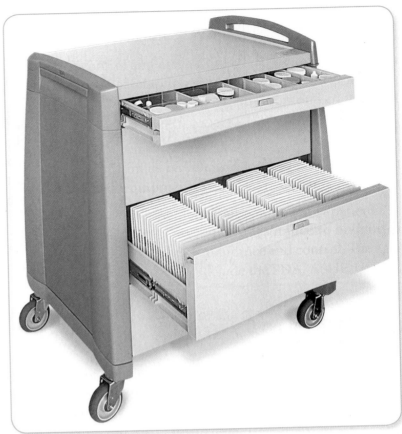

Figure 10-3 Unit-dose medication cart. (Courtesy of Artromick International, Inc.)

Usually, cassettes are filled every 24 hours, or once per shift, wit only those medications that the patient will need during the specified peric of time. Pharmacy personnel exchange unit doses for new medication when medication orders are changed. Most oral, injectable, and topic medications can be placed into the cassette drawers. Multi-dose vials a used for injectables that are not available in unit doses. These contain sever doses of medication instead of just one dose.

When filled cassettes are delivered to nursing stations, they a exchanged for previously used cassettes, which are returned to the pharma for restocking. A "fill list" is generated from the patient's profile, and t patient is only charged for the doses that are actually taken out of the casse drawers to be dispensed.

Accurate cassette filling and double-checking of medication conte is very important. The drug's correct name, strength, and dosage form m be verified before any administration occurs. Robotic systems are now us in many hospitals for unit-dose drug distribution to ensure accuracy combination with bar code technology.

Procedure: Filling Cassettes for Unit-Dose Distribution

Objective: To properly demonstrate the procedures for filling cassettes for unit-dose distribution.

Equipment Needed: fill list, unit-dose cassette, unit-dose medications

Step 1: Read the "fill list" of medications that has been verified by the pharmacist (Figure 10-4A).

Step 2: Remove the first unit-dose medication from stock (Figure 10-4B).

Step 3: Verify its name, strength, and dosage form.

Step 4: Place it in the patient's cassette (Figure 10-4C).

Step 5: Repeat the procedure for each required medication for this patient.

Step 6: Have another individual verify the filled cassette for accuracy.

Figure 10-4 Filling patient cassettes. (A) Review fill list (B) Choose correct unit dose medication (C) Place unit dose medication in the patient's cassette.

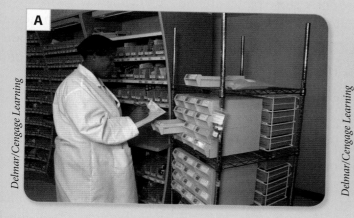

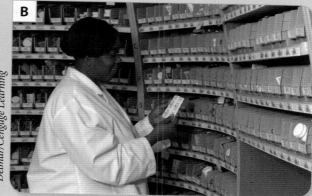

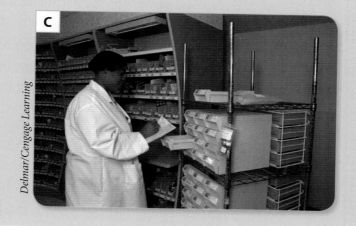

Exercise

Objective: To become familiar with the procedure for filling patient cassettes.

Practice filling cassettes accurately and double-checking all medications' names, strengths, and dosage forms.

DRUG STORAGE AND INVENTORY CONTROL

Inventory may be divided into an active drug inventory and a backup storeroom inventory, including division by how drugs will be used.

Storage

Drugs must be properly stored after they have been selected, ordered, and received. Proper storage requires security requirements, environmental considerations (proper temperature, ventilation, humidity, light, and sanitation), safety requirements, proper rotation, computerization, and turnover rate.

Security Requirements

Often, only authorized personnel can have access to certain drugs. Legend drugs must be dispensed by a licensed pharmacist, though pharmacy technicians who are supervised by a pharmacist can handle floor stock orders and deliver these medications to drug storage locations. Controlled (Schedule II) substances and certain alcohol can only be ordered, received, prepared, and dispensed by licensed pharmacists, with pharmacy technicians allowed to assist under direct supervision. Daily physical counts of inventory are essential to ensure no misuse of controlled substances.

Dangerous substances must be stored in cool, properly ventilated areas. Caustic substances should be stored in locked cabinets instead of open shelves. Anti-cancer agents should be sealed in protective outer bags to protect the immediate containers from breaking and coming into contact with pharmacy staff. Protective clothing also helps to ensure exposure to anti-cancer agents.

Proper Rotation of Inventory

Drugs should be separated by category, as the Joint Commission requires internal and external medications to be stored separately to reduce the potential for incorrect administration. By properly rotating inventory (including checking expiration dates upon receipt of new products), the potential for dispensing or administering expired drugs can be greatly reduced. Proper rotation also helps to ensure that most drugs are used before they become outdated.

Alert!

Drugs with expiration dates that are further away should always be stored on shelves behind drugs that have more imminent expiration dates.

Exercise

Objective: To become familiar with the proper storage procedures used in the pharmacy.

Select a shelf of empty drug containers and organize it so that those with the most imminent expiration dates are at the front of the shelf, and those with the longest time left before they expire are at the back.

Computerized Inventory Control

Computerized perpetual inventory systems are now in use to indicate when medications should be reordered. These systems also allow for each drug's monthly usage rate to be monitored and to determine which department is using which drug and at what rate. Computerized inventory control also helps to control budgets by determining trends of use and prescribing of medications.

Turnover Rate

A pharmacy's inventory turnover rate is calculated by dividing total dollars spent to purchase drugs for 1 year by the actual value of the inventory at any point in time. This shows how many times in a year the inventory has been used or replaced. Higher turnover rates have been noted since the establishment of prime vendor programs and computerized order-entry systems. Storerooms should be checked at regular intervals to verify that reorder points for medications are correct. Minimum and maximum inventories should be maintained, with proper space allotted to store each product. Inventories should be controlled not only in the pharmacy, but also in nursing units, emergency rooms, operating rooms, and recovery rooms.

SUMMARY

Pharmacy technicians play an important role in minimizing pharmacy operation costs by inventory control. Good inventory control allows the pharmacy to have enough pharmaceutical products on hand to fill prescriptions and orders for compounding without having so much stock that drugs expire before they can be used.

Pharmacy technicians must follow the policies and procedures of inventory control, provide accurate record keeping, receive and store pharmaceutical products, and remove all expired products from the shelves.

Pharmacies may purchase pharmaceutical products from different sources, including manufacturers, wholesalers, purchasing groups, prime vendors, and other pharmacies. Documenting receipts of inventory may be done by entering information into a computer, or by scanning bar codes.

Controlled substances require detailed record keeping because they have high abuse potential. The DEA has strict guidelines for ordering, receiving, storing, and destroying Schedule II through IV controlled substances.

Other important tasks for inventory control include drug distribution (in the hospital pharmacy), unit-dose distribution, proper rotation, and drug storage.

REVIEW QUESTIONS

Multiple Choice

1. Which of the following is *not* the responsibility of the pharmacy technician in inventory control?

   A. ordering and receiving controlled (Schedule II) drugs
   B. receiving and storing pharmaceutical products
   C. identifying and ordering needed pharmaceutical products
   D. following the policies and procedures of inventory control

2. Which of the following sources of pharmaceutical products offer the lowest price and requires a minimum-quantity order if the pharmacy purchases from them?

   A. prime vendors
   B. purchasing groups
   C. wholesalers
   D. manufacturers

3. Which of the following may be identified by a National Drug Code (NDC) number?

   A. drug product
   B. manufacturer's name
   C. drug dosage and strength
   D. all of the above

4. The pharmacy technician can keep track of drugs that are sold by listing them:

   A. in a "want book"
   B. in a computer system (by using their numeric identifiers)
   C. by using their bar codes
   D. all of the above

5. Which of the following has strict guidelines for ordering, receiving, or storing Schedule II through IV substances?

   A. FDA   C. DEA
   B. CDC   D. all of the above

6. Controlled substances are usually stored in which of the following pharmacy sites?

   A. stock shelves that are separate from other drug shelves
   B. locked area
   C. clean room
   D. pharmacy director's office

7. All of the following are advantages of unit-dose drug distribution systems, except:

   A. decreased drug abuse
   B. decreased pharmacy technician time
   C. decreased chance of medication errors
   D. decreased inventory of medications in the pharmacy

8. The volume of most IV piggybacks is which of the following?

   A. 50 to 100 mL of fluid   C. 750 to 1000 mL of fluid
   B. 250 to 500 mL of fluid   D. all of the above

9. Usually, cassettes are filled every:

   A. hour   C. 12 hours
   B. 6 hours   D. 24 hours

10. Inventories should be controlled in which of the following places?

    A. nursing units   C. emergency rooms
    B. operating rooms   D. all of the above

Fill in the Blank

1. The drug distribution system used in the pharmacy that involves individual medication packages is referred to as _____.

2. External medications must be stored _____ from internal medications in the pharmacy.

3. Only authorized personnel in the pharmacy can have _____ to certain drugs.

4. Most oral, injectable, and topical medications can be placed into the _____ drawers.

5. IV mixtures are prepared inside _____ within a clean room.

6. Chemotherapy drugs are usually kept in their own secured area of the pharmacy due to their _____.

7. An organized inventory system is also known as an _____ system.

8. Bar codes greatly simplify both _____ processes and sales.

9. Many medications are purchase by the pharmacy from a "prime vendor," which guarantees a lower _____.

10. A drug's _____ is based on its stability, and describes the length of time it can be kept in stock before its contents become altered.

Quality Control and Assurance

OUTLINE

OBJECTIVES

Upon completion of this chapter, the student should be able to:

1. Define quality control and assurance.
2. Explain why quality control is needed.
3. Explain the goals of quality improvement.
4. Discuss the three levels of ASHP guidelines.
5. Discuss the implications of USP Chapter <797>.
6. Explain the role of the Joint Commission in quality control.
7. Describe the publications of the AMA.

GLOSSARY

Admix – Mix or blend.

Alum – Aluminum sulfate; used to help boost immune response, as an emetic, or as an astringent or styptic (both of which cause contraction).

Audit – Examination or verification conducted to assure effectiveness and correctness.

Contamination – Containing unwanted substances or organisms.

Turbidity – Muddiness created by stirring up sediment or having foreign particles suspended.

OVERVIEW

Quality control and assurance is designed to achieve the utmost quality, purity, effectiveness, and safety concerning drug products. The Food and Drug Administration (FDA) has issued many guidelines overseeing specific dosage forms and operations that include aseptic manufacturing, stability testing, and validation. Quality system inspections are a regular part of regulatory pre-approval programs for new drugs.

Inadequate quality control practices may lead to contamination of pharmaceuticals as well as medication errors. The pharmacy is responsible for the storage of all pharmaceuticals, for monitoring expiration dates, and for monitoring the temperature of refrigerators and freezers used to store pharmaceuticals.

Pharmacy technicians and other pharmacy staff must understand the importance of quality control and assurance when dealing with sterile pharmaceutical compounding. They must ensure integrity of the process and the final product. Poor quality control may result in a potential risk and harm to patient and personnel.

POLICIES AND PROCEDURES FOR QUALITY CONTROL AND ASSURANCE

Pharmacy technicians must follow the policies and procedures of the workplace in regard to quality control and assurance. The director of pharmacy writes the quality and control policies and procedures for all personnel to follow. Those who deal with sterile compounding are required to have in-depth training and an appropriate academic education.

Policies and procedures that relate to quality control and assurance include the following areas:

- Acquisition, Handling, and Storage.

  - Acquisition – dating of bulk drug substances; guidelines for repackaging; systems for purchasing equipment and other supplies; testing ingredients in order to identify them; and USP NF standards for selection of ingredients.

  - Handling – ampule and vial decontamination; anteroom activities (such as removing outer packaging); disposal of hazardous or used equipment and items; handling of supplies contained in pouches; inspection of sterile containers and ingredients before compounding; the quarantining or removing of expired drugs and supplies; and the recall procedures for specific preparations.

- Storage – inspection and rotation of stock; proper location of quarantined preparations; standards for exposure to humidity, light, or ventilation; and temperature monitoring.

- Beyond-use Dating – the determining of stabilities of preparations; experimental testing for stability; handling those preparations removed or returned to refrigeration; how to set beyond-use dates; and setting expiration times as related to specific storage temperatures.

- Environmental Monitoring – the development of a plan to monitor clean room air, ceilings, floors, surfaces, and walls; periodic monitoring of air particulates; sampling air and surfaces for microbes; specifications for monitoring devices.

- Equipment – calibration of equipment; cleaning and using equipment and fixtures; sterilizing nonsterile equipment; where carts, equipment, and supplies should be located; use of, traffic near, and cleaning of laminar-airflow hoods or workbenches; and the use of automatic compounding devices and pumps.

- Facilities – cleaning work areas, controlling traffic, the types of preparations that may be compounded, and safety equipment.

- Labeling – batch preparations, patient-use preparations, routine order preparations, and storage of labels.

- Personnel Behavior – eating, drinking, and smoking areas; hand washing and drying; dealing with personnel who have infectious conditions; exposure protection; and what may be worn in the clean room and under airflow hoods.

- Personnel Training and Evaluation – aseptic technique; basic educational requirements; competencies; compounding practices; equipment operation; handling of preparations; job orientation; physical requirements; responsibilities of employees; training on drug properties; and working conditions.

- Preparation – aseptic technique; batch compounding records; inspection of ingredients and containers; master work sheets; pharmaceutical standards and references; and standards of compatibility, physiology, purity, and stability.

- Protective Equipment – donning and removing garments; re-use of garments; use of gloves, hair covers, masks, and shoe covers; use of adhesive mats to clean shoes.

- Sterilization – methods for sterilization; quarantine and release procedures; and sterile filtration procedures.

- Validation of Processes – competence of staff members for each type of preparation; reevaluation of competencies and processes.

FACTORS INFLUENCING QUALITY CONTROL AND ASSURANCE

There must be a documented and continuing quality assurance control program in place to monitor personnel performance, equipment, and facilities. Appropriate samples of finished products must be examined to assure that the pharmacy is capable of consistently preparing sterile pharmaceuticals to meet specifications.

Improper aseptic technique can lead to **contamination** of pharmaceuticals. Before preparing sterile products, you should always:

- Perform hand and forearm hygiene, using a detergent or antimicrobial soap, or by using an alcohol skin hygiene product.

- Wipe or spray the rubber stoppers of containers with 70% alcohol.

- Disinfect all surfaces of ampules, vials, and container closures prior to entering a laminar-airflow hood.

- Avoid touching sterile supplies until proper personal protective equipment has been donned.

It is important to remember that no eating, drinking, or smoking is allowed in the sterile preparation area. Contaminated multi-dose vials (MDVs) may cause infections. When they are used, they should be refrigerated after opening. The rubber diaphragm of the vial should be cleaned with alcohol before any usage, and touch contamination should be avoided before the diaphragm is penetrated. MDVs should be discarded when empty or if possible contamination has occurred.

Inadequate quality control can lead to contamination. Steps for preventing contamination of pharmaceuticals include:

- **Admixed** parenterals should be stored in a refrigerator beginning immediately after preparation (usually for up to 1 week).

- All admixed parenteral should be labeled according to ASHP recommendations.

- Batch-prepared items should be labeled with lot numbers included.

- Sterile products should be checked for cracks, leaks, **turbidity**, or particulate matter (which can indicate contamination).

Exercise

Objective: To become familiar with the process of checking drugs for contaminants and expiration dates.

Remove 10 sample admixtures that have been stored in a refrigerator and check them for cracks, leaks, turbidity. Also check their expiration dates. Properly discard those that are expired, damaged, or no longer visibly clear.

MEDICATION ERRORS

Though the incidence of medication errors is actually only a fraction of the millions of prescriptions and doses prepared yearly, even one error is too many. There should be zero tolerance for medication errors. Accuracy must be strived for at all times regardless of the drug product or procedure. Check-and-balance systems are in place in all settings that help to avoid medication errors. Most errors occur within the drug use process, and are usually caused by a failure of the system rather than the failure of one person. Adverse drug reactions, allergic drug reactions, drug-drug interactions, and medication errors are commonly referred to as *drug misadventures* or *adverse drug events*.

Exercise

Objective: To become aware of common medication errors.

List 5 factors that are related to medication errors.

QUALITY IMPROVEMENT

Quality improvement strives to achieve continued quality over time. Correct training, up-to-date equipment and facilities, and proper facilities management serve to assure that continued quality improvement is implemented. The close evaluation of all procedures and even individual steps helps to minimize errors of any sort. Check-and-balance systems should be continuously monitored and revised. Regular **audits** of personnel, equipment, facilities, policies, and procedures can help to identify problem areas (or those that may be developing) so that corrective measures can be taken.

Written procedures, end-product testing, formal operator training, equipment maintenance, and process checkpoints are all essential in maintaining quality control as well as quality assurance. Quality assurance process checkpoints may include double-checking of:

- The drug and dosage form being repackaged.

- The expiration date of the bulk product being used.

- Fill volumes, and how they relate to the proper dose and proper container.

- Calculations used for reconstituting drug products.

- Information (including spelling) located on labels, computers, and any stencils that are being used.

Alert!

The quality assurance process must identify problems or areas for improvement of patient care.

Agency Guidelines for Quality Assurance

Below, the various guidelines used for quality assurance are listed individually for each important agency. These guidelines help to ensure universal testing and standard practices for quality assurance and control.

Food and Drug Administration

The FDA revises their Good Manufacturing Practices (GMP) on a regular basis. The GMP oversees quality compounding of sterile products, and other FDA documents focus on aseptic processing of sterile products, with proper standards in place that must be met. The current GMP regulations and additional guidelines should be understood thoroughly by those involved in pursuing quality control and quality assurance responsibilities. The FDA's Office of New Drug Quality Assessment (ONDQA) assesses quality attributes and the manufacturing of new drugs. It also sets standards to assure safety and efficacy of new drugs, and safe development of new drugs.

When medications are prepared or compounded, the FDA requires that steps be taken to avoid contamination, including sterile technique, clean rooms, airflow hoods, and the visual inspection of all medications being used (to check for contamination). Class 100 environments, including that provided by laminar-airflow hoods, are required for intravenous admixtures, sterile products that are made from nonsterile ingredients, and those mixtures that will not be administered within 24 hours.

> **Alert!**
>
> *Federal standards are currently not enforced for environmental quality, but guidance is available in the FDA Concept Paper.*

American Society of Health System Pharmacists

The American Society of Health System Pharmacists (ASHP) addresses quality assurance on a wide basis. They focus on many different areas, including sterile products, other types of pharmaceuticals, and testing of products. Their publication, the *ASHP Guidelines on Quality Assurance for Pharmacy Prepared Sterile Products,* addresses all areas affected by quality assurance.

Risk Levels from ASHP Guidelines

There are three risk levels in the ASHP Guidelines on Quality Assurance for Pharmacy-Prepared Sterile Products, as follows:

- Level 1 – Includes products to be stored at room temperature and administered completely within 28 hours after being prepared; unpreserved, sterile products that are prepared for more than one patient that contain preservatives; or products prepared by closed-system aseptic transfer of nonpyrogenic, sterile, finished products (in sterile containers) from licensed manufacturers. These include:
  - Single-patient admixtures.
  - Sterile ophthalmics.

- Syringes without preservatives used within 28 hours.

- Batch-prefilled syringes with preservatives.

- TPN solutions made by gravity transfer of carbohydrates and amino acids with addition of sterile additives.

- Level 2 – Includes products administered more than 28 hours after preparation and stored at room temperature; products that are batch-prepared with no preservatives for more than one patient; products compounded by various manipulations of sterile ingredients using closed-system aseptic transfer from licensed manufacturers. These include:

  - Injections to be used in a portable pump or reservoir over several days.

  - Batch-reconstituted antibiotics without preservatives.

  - Batch-prefilled syringes without preservatives.

  - TPN solutions mixed with automatic compounding devices.

- Level 3 – Includes products compounded from nonsterile components, containers, or equipment before they are terminally sterilized; products prepared with sterile or nonsterile ingredients using open-system transfer before they are terminally sterilized. These include:

  - **Alum** bladder irrigations.

  - Morphine injections made from powders or tablets.

  - TPN solutions made from dry amino acids or sterilized by final filtration.

  - Autoclaved IV solutions.

USP <797>

United States Pharmacopeia (USP) Chapter <797> is the first (enforceable) set of standards defining many quality control areas. Along with the ASHP guidelines, USP <797> lists all necessary quality control processes. This includes quality control risk levels, personnel, education, evaluation, policies, procedures, storage, handling, facilities, equipment, aseptic technique, product preparation, garb, process validation, and evaluation of end-products.

The Joint Commission on Accreditation of Healthcare Organizations

The Joint Commission publishes standards for the control of pharmaceuticals and companies that manufacture, store, and deliver them. The Joint Commission standards are regularly reevaluated and revised based upon stringent inspection techniques. The Joint Commission also accredits health care organizations to ensure high standards of patient care. It also acts to help organizations to become accredited.

Center for Drug Evaluation and Research

The Center for Drug Evaluation and Research (CDER) assures that safe and effective drugs are available in the United States. It initially sought to improve the controls set forth in the Pure Food and Drug Act of 1906. Drug evaluation and approval for marketing is the CDER's primary activity. It is the responsibility of the CDER to determine whether the benefits of a drug outweigh its risks. The CDER classifies New Drug Applications (NDAs) according to the type of drug and its intended uses. It also conducts onsite inspections of manufacturing sites, and holds clinical trials to verify the completeness of drug information, accuracy of data, good manufacturing controls, standards compliances, and the collection of samples for drug analysis.

American Medical Association

The mission of the American Medical Association (AMA) is to promote the art and science of medicine for the betterment of public health, to advance the interests of physicians and their patients, to promote public health, to lobby for favorable legislation, and to raise money for medical education. It has a *council on drugs*, which focuses on the field of pharmacy and the process of drug manufacturing and resultant effects on public health. The AMA publishes the *Journal of the American Medical Association* (*JAMA*), as well as many other documents, including *Drug Evaluations*, which evaluates and compares different drug therapies.

Centers for Disease Control and Prevention

The guidelines established by the Centers for Disease Control and Prevention (CDC) are important to use in the prevention of disease and infection. They provide invaluable information about aseptic technique and various environmental controls designed to prevent infection. The CDC places consistent emphasis on emerging infectious diseases and conducts research to help prevent their spread.

ROLE OF THE PHARMACY TECHNICIAN

Pharmacy technicians must understand the concept of the necessity of quality control and assurance. They must be involved with environmental control and monitoring, quality testing of compounded dosage forms, evaluation of personnel aseptic technique, various steps of quality assurance, determination of risk levels of various products, standard operating procedures, personnel training and competency, storage, and beyond-use dating.

The pharmacy technician should be familiar with various agency guidelines for quality assurance, including those set forth by the FDA, ASHP, Joint Commission, CDC, and AMA. Quality control and assurance are responsibilities of pharmacy technicians. They may involve all of the following:

- Making sure there are no expired medications in the pharmacy.
- Making sure that refrigerators and freezers are at appropriate temperatures.
- Maintaining a daily log of the temperatures.
- Avoiding contamination in compounding products.
- Making sure that medication errors do not occur.

SUMMARY

The goal of quality control and assurance is to achieve the utmost quality, purity, effectiveness, and safety concerning drug products. Inadequate quality control practices can result in medication errors and contamination.

Pharmacy technicians must check expiration dates and monitor temperature of refrigerator and freezers used to store pharmaceuticals. Quality assurance control must be documented to monitor personnel performance, facilities, and equipment. Sterile pharmaceuticals and aseptic technique must be met.

The various guidelines used for quality assurance to help universal testing and standard practices for quality assurance and control. The agencies that regulate or suggest these guidelines include the FDA, ASHP, USP <797>, Joint Commission, and CDER.

REVIEW QUESTIONS

Multiple Choice

1. Which of the following was the first enforceable national published standard for sterile compounding of drugs?

   A. USP <797>   **C.** HIPAA
   B. JCAHO   **D.** CDC

2. Which of the following standards are regularly reevaluated and revised based upon stringent inspection techniques?

   A. USP <797>   **C.** HIPAA
   B. JCAHO   **D.** CDC

3. Which of the following agencies assures that safe and effective drugs are available in the United States?

   A. Joint Commission on Accreditation of Healthcare Organizations
   B. Centers for Disease Control and Prevention
   C. American Medical Association
   D. Center for Drug Evaluation and Research

4. Contaminated multi-dose vials may cause:

   A. turbidity   **C.** infection
   B. infestation   **D.** infarction

5. Which of the following factors cause medication errors?

   A. pharmacy technicians, during dispensing and calculation
   B. nurses, during administration of medications
   C. physicians, while ordering medications
   D. all of the above

6. Which of the following oversees quality compounding of sterile products?

   A. FDA
   B. ASHP
   C. JCAHO
   D. CDER

7. Which of the following organizations is responsible for the accreditation of pharmaceutical manufacturers?

   A. FDA
   B. ASHP
   C. JCAHO
   D. CDC

8. Which of the following organizations promotes the art and science of medicine for the betterment of public health?

   A. JCAHO
   B. CDER
   C. ASHP
   D. AMA

9. Examinations or verifications conducted to assure effectiveness and correctness are known as:

   A. enforcement
   B. audits
   C. attuning
   D. attendance

10. Inadequate quality control can lead to:

    A. medication errors
    B. contamination
    C. health risks
    D. all of the above

Fill in the Blank

1. All admixed parenterals should be labeled according to _____ recommendations.

2. USP <797> lists all necessary _____ processes.

3. Appropriate samples of finished products must be examined to assure that the _____ is capable of consistently preparing _____ pharmaceuticals to meet specifications.

4. Disinfect all surfaces of ampules, vials, and container closure prior to entering a _____ hood.

5. It is important to remember that no eating, drinking, or smoking is allowed in the _____ preparation area.

6. Admixed parenterals should be stored in a _____ beginning immediately after preparation.

7. All admixed parenterals should be _____ according to ASHP recommendations.

8. According to the ASHP Guidelines on Quality Assurance for pharmacy preparation of sterile products, there are _____ risk levels.

9. The rubber diaphragm of a vial should be cleaned with _____ before any usage.

10. _____ should be checked for cracks, leaks, turbidity, or particulate matter, which can indicate contamination.

SELF-EVALUATION

Test for General Concepts

Multiple Choice

1. Which of the following characterizes the various types of compounding?

    A. Each type has its own unique focus and specialization.
    B. Each type can be done without a prescription.
    C. Each type has its own risks of contamination.
    D. both A and C

2. Nuclear pharmacy compounding focuses on:

    A. daily intravenous medications
    B. radiopharmaceuticals
    C. total parenteral nutrition solutions
    D. none of the above

3. Which of the following is a part of the Department of Labor?

    A. the Joint Commission
    B. OSHA
    C. HIPAA
    D. none of the above

4. Radiation safety standards are established by which of the following?

    A. the national board of pharmacy
    B. the Occupational Safety and Health Administration
    C. the state boards of pharmacy
    D. the CDC

5. When a staff member discovers a fire before the fire alarm has sounded, he or she should first make an attempt to do which of the following?

    A. call the director of the pharmacy
    B. call 911
    C. extinguish the fire
    D. exit the building immediately

6. Exits must be marked and escape routes published on:

   A. an OSHA poster
   B. a fire safety plan
   C. an exposure control plan
   D. a hazard communication plan

7. Any Schedule II drug that has been dropped or spilled requires which of the following?

   A. notification of the supervisor
   B. proper equipment and devices
   C. proper skills in dealing with any accident
   D. proper documentation of the accident to be completed

8. Which of the following terms means "increasing the action of another drug"?

   A. systemic action
   B. synergistic action
   C. selective action
   D. microbial action

9. All of the following are universal precautions, except:

   A. wearing jewelry during compounding IV admixtures
   B. wearing personal protective equipment
   C. using a sharps container to contain used needles
   D. appropriately handling chemotherapy agents

10. Which of the following is an example of selective drug action?

    A. depressants
    B. antimicrobials
    C. topicals, for local effects
    D. all of the above

11. Which of the following regulates all workplaces by enforcing the proper removal of hazards, and the use of emergency plans?

    A. HIPAA
    B. the Joint Commission
    C. OSHA
    D. all of the above

12. Implantable devices placed beneath the skin near blood vessels that lie beneath may be used:

    A. for contraception
    B. to treat cancer
    C. to treat diabetes
    D. to treat angina pectoris

13. Adhesive patches transfer a drug through the skin, and are commonly used:

    A. to treat angina pectoris
    B. for smoking cessation
    C. to treat motion sickness
    D. all of the above

14. Prescription drugs are also called:

  A. legal drugs
  B. legend drugs
  C. routine prescriptions
  D. over-the-counter drugs

15. All of the following factors may influence increasing pharmaceutical compounding activities, except:

  A. shortages of drug products and combinations
  B. special patient populations
  C. a varying number of dosage forms
  D. a limited number of drug strengths

16. The preparation, mixing, assembling, packaging, and labeling of a drug is referred to as:

  A. dispensing
  B. compounding
  C. sorting
  D. selecting

17. Routine prescriptions are also known as:

  A. standing orders
  B. hospital drug charts
  C. batch-prepared prescriptions
  D. maintenance prescriptions

18. Which of the following products is typically compounded by a hospital pharmacy?

  A. radiopharmaceuticals
  B. total parenteral nutrition
  C. both A and B
  D. none of the above

19. Many compounded drugs, which are reconstituted, have a beyond-use date ranging between 30 days and:

  A. 3 months
  B. 6 months
  C. 8 months
  D. 12 months

20. A master formula sheet contains which of the following information?

  A. the ingredients of a formulation
  B. the manufacturer's expiration date
  C. the date it was prepared
  D. all of the above

21. The length of time that a drug remains potent is referred to as its:

  A. shelf life
  B. date of expiration
  C. date of dispensing
  D. dosage

22. Which of the following professional people are responsible to select the most appropriate chemicals to use for compounding?

    A. physicians
    B. pharmacists
    C. pharmacy technicians
    D. all of the above

23. Which of the following will the pharmacy technician work with when compounding?

    A. intravenous minibags
    B. large-volume parenteral admixtures
    C. unit-dose injections
    D. all of the above

24. Which of the following is the most effective method to decrease the risk of infection for pharmacy technicians?

    A. standard precautions
    B. immunizations
    C. medications
    D. personal hygiene

25. All equipment for emergency drugs and supplies should be checked on a regular basis for functionality and freshness. This should occur:

    A. daily
    B. weekly
    C. monthly
    D. both B and C

26. Which of the following actions is more appropriate to prevent latex allergy?

    A. wearing powder-free gloves
    B. wearing doubled gloves
    C. doing allergy tests
    D. none of the above

27. If an object is stable and has handles, which of the following amounts of weight is considered the heaviest amount that can be safely lifted?

    A. 21 pounds
    B. 31 pounds
    C. 41 pounds
    D. 51 pounds

28. Which of the following is a simple but very important step in preventing the transmission of bloodborne pathogens?

    A. wearing gloves
    B. up-to-date immunizations
    C. hand washing
    D. wearing gowns

29. Most retail pharmacies store their medications alphabetically by:

    A. generic name
    B. chemical name
    C. brand name
    D. manufacturer's name

30. The majority of drugs are stored:

    A. in a refrigerator
    B. in a freezer
    C. at room temperature
    D. in none of the above ways

31. Which of the following agencies considers non-prescription drugs safe enough to use without a physician's advice?

    A. the DEA
    B. the FDA
    C. the Joint Commission
    D. OSHA

32. All of the following drugs are common OTC products except:

    A. ibuprofen and aspirin
    B. herbal supplements
    C. penicillins
    D. vitamins

33. The United States Pharmacopoeia/National Formulary book is updated every:

    A. 2 years
    B. 3 years
    C. 4 years
    D. 5 years

34. Losses of controlled substances first must be reported to the local office of the:

    A. DEA
    B. CDC
    C. FDA
    D. police department

35. The pink section of the Physician's Desk Reference (PDR) lists which of the following?

    A. brand names and generic names
    B. product information
    C. alphabetical arrangement by drug manufacturer
    D. classifications of drugs

36. All controlled substance are listed in the PDR with:

    A. the symbol B
    B. the symbol G
    C. the symbol C
    D. none of the above

37. Which of the following medications usually reverses most occurrences of anaphylaxis?

    A. morphine
    B. oxygen
    C. Benadryl
    D. epinephrine

38. Which of the following routes of drug administration reaches the systemic circulation rapidly?

    A. sublingual
    B. oral
    C. rectal
    D. none of the above

39. Which of the following drug reference books is more up-to-date and comprehensive than the others?

    A. the Physician's Desk Reference
    B. Drug Facts and Comparisons
    C. the United States Pharmacopoeia – Drug Information
    D. all of the them are the same

40. Expiration dates should be checked carefully before:

    A. being dispensed
    B. being compounded
    C. being administered
    D. all of the above

Fill in the Blank

1. If you know the brand name of a drug, located in the pink section of the PDR, you can then easily find the _____ name.

2. Ambulatory care compounding is designed for patients who do not require a _____ _____.

3. A master formula sheet may be used to document information about each _____ that is used in the pharmacy.

4. The process of a drug passing into body fluids and tissues by means of diffusion is known as _____.

5. Compounding pharmacists use chemicals that come from reliable commercial sources that are _____ by various governmental _____.

6. Nuclear pharmacy compounding focuses on radioactive drugs that are used for _____ or _____.

7. Stability may be chemical, _____, or microbiological.

8. For sterile products, a clean air environment consisting of laminar-airflow hoods and isolation barriers must be used, except in an _____.

9. Eye wash stations must be available for flushing _____ from the eyes.

10. Most ambulatory patients are responsible for obtaining and _____ their own medications.

11. When a pharmacy technician prepares, compounds, or dispenses medications, care must be taken to _____.

12. Biohazard symbols should be displayed on specific _____.

13. Piggybacks and large-volume parenteral nutrition admixtures may also be involved with _____ injections and total parenteral nutrition solutions.

14. Compounding means the preparation, _____, _____, _____, or _____ of a drug or device as the result of a practitioner's prescription.

15. The degree of pathogenicity of a pathogen is referred to as _____.

Matching

1. _____ Preventing transmission of infection

2. _____ Systemic hypersensitivity

3. _____ Can be affected by an agent

4. _____ A fine mist containing minute particles

5. _____ Narrowing of the blood vessels

    A. Vasoconstrictor
    B. Host
    C. Anaphylaxis
    D. Aerosolization
    E. Isolation

Test for Nonsterile Compounding Products

Multiple Choice

1. Which of the following is an advantage of both single-unit and single-dose packages?

   A. reduction of the need for pharmacy technicians to repackage medications from manufacturers
   B. reduction of medication prices
   C. increased medication errors
   D. all of the above

2. Which of the following is a disadvantage of using glass containers over plastic containers?

   A. transparency
   B. they are reusable
   C. weight
   D. they may be heated

3. Appropriate storage of compounding products requires which of the following factors?

   A. security issues
   B. safety
   C. environmental considerations
   D. all of the above

4. Which of the following equipment is used to pick up prescription weights?

   A. pestles
   B. counter balances
   C. forceps
   D. compounding slabs

5. Spring-based Class A balances have a weighing capacity that ranges from:

   A. 3 mg to 42 grams
   B. 6 mg to 90 grams
   C. 6 mg to 120 grams
   D. 60 grams to 5 kilograms

6. Simple liquid containers that may be cylindrical in shape are known as:

   A. beakers
   B. droppers
   C. funnels
   D. graduates

7. A type of suspension that consists of two different liquids that are held together by a specific agent is known as:

   A. a gel
   B. an elixir
   C. an emulsion
   D. a magma

8. Which of the following are generally calibrated in metric units (cubic centimeters)?

   A. droppers
   B. graduates
   C. pipettes
   D. all of the above

9. To grind a powder into a smoother mixture, using moisture, is a process called:

   A. pasteurization
   B. agitation
   C. suspension
   D. levigation

10. Which of the following dosage forms is prepared by the heat method?

    A. syrups
    B. emulsions
    C. suspensions
    D. elixirs

11. When the size of a capsule is "number 2," what is the approximate amount contained?

    A. 400 mg
    B. 300 mg
    C. 150 mg
    D. 100 mg

12. Which of the following dosage forms can be used when patients have difficulty in swallowing?

    A. caplets
    B. capsules
    C. tablets
    D. powders

13. Which term means "reducing to a fine powder by grinding"?

    A. trituration
    B. suspending
    C. agitation
    D. atomization

14. Which of the following is the appropriate method for mixing two different powders?

    A. The lighter powder should be placed on top of the heavier powder and then blended.
    B. The heavier powder should be placed on top of the lighter powder and then blended.
    C. It can be done either way.
    D. It is not possible to mix two different types of powders.

15. Dry baths allow both cooling and heating, with commonly available temperatures as low as:

    A. –30 degrees Centigrade
    B. –20 degrees Centigrade
    C. –10 degrees Centigrade
    D. 0 degrees Centigrade

16. Which of the following items may be easily cleaned with alcohol?

    A. crimpers
    B. decappers
    C. beakers
    D. all of the above

17. How often must freezers be checked?

    A. at least every day
    B. at least every week
    C. at least every month
    D. at least every 6 months

18. Which of the following is the largest capsule size?

    A. 000
    B. 00
    C. 0
    D. 1

19. Brushes may be designed for which of the following sciences?

    A. cytology
    B. microbiology
    C. both A and B
    D. none of the above

20. Which of the following devices are used to seal vials and other containers with caps?

    A. crimpers
    B. tongs
    C. brushes
    D. beakers

21. Master formula sheets are also referred to as:

    A. insurance records
    B. medical order records
    C. bulk compounding formula records
    D. none of the above

22. Which of the following are ideal for preparing samples of flexible packaging materials?

    A. drying racks
    B. dry baths
    C. hot plates
    D. heat sealers

23. Which of the following are not semisolid drugs?

    A. pastes
    B. creams
    C. lozenges
    D. ointments

24. Diluents used in tablet compounding are usually mixtures of:

    A. lactose, sucrose, ethyl alcohol, and water
    B. glycogen, glucose, and water
    C. maltose, sucrose, and ethyl alcohol
    D. lactose, maltose, methyl alcohol, and water

25. Which of the following numbers is the largest oral size capsule that is suitable for most patients?

    A. 000
    B. 00
    C. 0
    D. 5

26. Inhaled powders are still commonly used to treat which of the following conditions?

    A. fever
    B. headaches
    C. hypertension
    D. nausea

27. Lozenges are also referred to as:

    A. powders
    B. pills
    C. pastes
    D. troches

28. Which of the following expiration dates is usually required for pharmaceutical drugs stored in the hospital pharmacy?

    A. 1 month
    B. 2 months
    C. 3 months
    D. 6 months

29. Which of the following can be used as an ointment base?

    A. oil-in-water emulsions
    B. water-in-oil emulsions
    C. absorption and water-soluble bases
    D. all of the above

30. Pastes are different from ointments, creams, and gels because:

    A. They contain a higher content of solids.
    B. They contain a lower content of solids.
    C. They are compounded in a different manner than ointments.
    D. none of the above

31. Topical drugs that have an oil base are called:

    A. creams
    B. ointments
    C. blisters
    D. all of the above

32. Which of the following is the reason that repackaging and labeling is required?

    A. when dosage forms are expensive
    B. when dosage forms are expired
    C. when dosage forms are not available
    D. all of the above

33. Which of the following bases is used for compounding suppositories?

    A. cocoa butter
    B. polyethylene glycol
    C. glycerinated gelatin
    D. all of the above

34. Which of the following are the simplest dosage forms compounded extemporaneously?

    A. solutions
    B. suspensions
    C. emulsions
    D. elixirs

35. Which of the following must be shaken well before being administered?

    A. solutions
    B. suspensions
    C. emulsions
    D. elixirs

36. Compounding slabs are usually made of:

    A. wood
    B. aluminum
    C. stainless steel
    D. ground glass

37. A liquid's concave surface, which results from surface tension, is known as its:

    A. viscosity
    B. gauge
    C. meniscus
    D. none of the above

38. Oil-in-water mixtures are usually used for which of the following routes of administration?

    A. oral
    B. topical
    C. both A and B
    D. none of the above

39. The two-pan type of Class A prescription balance requires external weights for measurements exceeding:

   A. 1 mg
   B. 10 mg
   C. 1 g
   D. 10 g

40. Which of the following is used underneath substances to be weighted to keep them from soiling balance pans?

   A. legal paper
   B. glassine paper
   C. wrapping paper
   D. aluminum foil

41. Suppository molds may be made of:

   A. plastic
   B. aluminum
   C. very hard rubber
   D. all of the above

42. Which of the following stirring rods have a flattened end that may also be used as a scoop?

   A. polypropylene
   B. rubber
   C. glass
   D. bendable Teflon

43. Which of the following is the correct option when repackaged pharmaceuticals expire?

   A. They must be returned to the manufacturer.
   B. They must be disposed of.
   C. They must be dispensed to patients quickly.
   D. They must be sent to third world countries.

44. All of the following medications cannot be divided into unit doses, except:

   A. metered-dose inhalers
   B. eye drops
   C. liquid medications
   D. creams

45. For accuracy, which of the following graduates should always be used to measure a certain volume of liquid?

   A. the smallest available that will hold the required volume
   B. the largest available that will hold the required volume
   C. a standard, medium-sized graduate
   D. none of the above

46. Table triturate molds are made of:

   A. glass
   B. wood
   C. metal
   D. ceramic

47. Which of the following are the most commonly dispensed repackaged types of medications in institutions?

    A. oral solids
    B. liquid injections
    C. semisolid drugs
    D. all of the above

48. Which of the following are especially useful for administering medications to infants?

    A. beakers
    B. funnels
    C. droppers
    D. stirring rods

49. Which of the following types of equipment is commonly used in conjunction with filter papers in order to remove insoluble particles?

    A. brushes
    B. pipettes
    C. blenders
    D. funnels

50. Beaker tongs are usually made of:

    A. stainless steel
    B. glass
    C. wood
    D. ceramic

Fill in the Blank

1. Making medications for individual patients is referred to as _____ compounding.

2. Many _____ of pharmacy have a required minimum list of equipment for compounding prescriptions.

3. Digital (electronic) Class A balances have a weighing capacity that ranges from _____ to a maximum of _____.

4. _____ is commonly used to clean balances after each procedure.

5. Gels that have large particle sizes in a two-phase system are referred to as _____.

6. Capsule shells are usually made of hard _____.

7. A _____ is a cup-shaped vessel in which materials are ground or crushed by a _____ in the preparation of drugs.

8. Certain emulsions must be compounded using _____ and porcelain mortars and pestles because glass mortars and pestles will not allow the formation of stable emulsions.

9. An instrument in the shape of a rod with one end that is rounded and weighted, used for crushing and mixing substances, is called a _____.

10. Ointments are most useful for the treatment of dermatologic conditions that include symptoms such as _____ skin.

11. An emulsion is a type of _____ that consists of two different liquids and an emulsifying agent that holds them together.

12. Spatulas are available in stainless steel, _____, or _____.

13. Glassine paper is available in either _____ or rectangular shapes.

14. Brushes may be made from natural or synthetic _____ materials.

15. _____ are used for sterile grasping and maneuvering of a variety of different types of laboratory equipment.

16. Weighing boats are used more frequently today than _____.

17. _____ are used to reduce particle size, usually for injectable products where particle size is essential.

18. Federal law requires that the expiration dates of repackaged drugs be _____ or less.

19. Manually operated oral solid repackaging systems are used for both blister and _____ packaging.

20. Manual capsule-filling systems are still used, usually 100 to _____ capsules at a time.

Matching

1. _____ Consists of two different liquids and an emulsifying agent.

2. _____ Grinding a powder into a smoother mixture using moisture.

3. _____ Consists of a very strong and impervious spun polythene.

4. _____ Contains solid drug particles floating in a liquid medium; easy to compound; must be shaken.

5. _____ A drug packaging that consists of clear plastic bags which are sealed with an adhesive.

6. _____ A small, medicated "candy" intended to be dissolved slowly within the mouth.

7. _____ A device used to measure liquids.

8. _____ An instrument that is rod-shaped, with one end that is rounded and weighted.

    A. Graduate
    B. Pestle
    C. Tyvek
    D. Pouch
    E. Levigation
    F. Lozenge
    G. Suspension
    H. Emulsion

Multiple Choice

1. Inventory control involves:

   A. maintaining an adequate savings account in the pharmacy setting
   B. maintaining an adequate stock of medications
   C. maintaining adequate continuing education for pharmacy technicians
   D. storing medications at nursing stations on each floor

2. Which of the following is a true statement?

   A. Most medications become more poisonous over time.
   B. All drugs must be sold regardless of their expiration dates.
   C. All drugs can lose value before their expiration dates.
   D. Most medications become less effective over time.

3. All of the following are common viral infections, except:

   A. measles
   B. herpes
   C. hypertrichosis
   D. chickenpox

4. Laminar-airflow hoods must be certified every:

   A. 2 months
   B. 6 months
   C. 12 months
   D. 2 years

5. Which of the following balances can weigh objects between 650 mg and 120 g?

   A. triple beam
   B. electronic balances
   C. Class A
   D. Class B

6. Which of the following should not be included by the pharmacy technician on a returned goods form?

   A. item number
   B. quality assurance
   C. quantity
   D. original purchase order number

7. Which of the following components of medical aseptic technique may reduce microbes?

    A. using sterile gloves
    B. proper cleaning of equipment
    C. regular hand washing
    D. all of the above

8. Outdated tetracycline has been shown to cause damage to which of the following body organs?

    A. bones
    B. lungs
    C. kidneys
    D. liver and gallbladder

9. A direct purchase is one that is made directly by the pharmacy from:

    A. the manufacturer
    B. the dealer
    C. another local pharmacy
    D. any of the above

10. Disposable syringes are available in a variety of sizes, that range from less than 1 mL to over:

    A. 20 mL
    B. 30 mL
    C. 40 mL
    D. 50 mL

11. Improper aseptic technique can lead to which of the following?

    A. administration of the wrong medications
    B. contamination of pharmaceuticals
    C. destruction of microorganisms
    D. all of the above

12. Admixed parenterals should be stored in a refrigerator for no longer than:

    A. 1 day
    B. 2 days
    C. 5 days
    D. 1 week

13. When orders of controlled substances arrive, they must be signed by the:

    A. nurse
    B. pharmacy technician
    C. pharmacist
    D. all of the above

14. Which of the following solutions should be used to clean a laminar-airflow hood?

    A. 70% rubbing alcohol
    B. 70% isopropyl alcohol
    C. 70% methyl alcohol
    D. 10% bleach

15. Needles come in various lengths, ranging from ¼ inch to:

   A. 1 inch
   B. 2 inches
   C. 3 inches
   D. 12 inches

16. Chemotherapy drugs are usually kept in their own secured area of the pharmacy due to their:

   A. cost
   B. toxicity
   C. quality
   D. quantity

17. Which of the following is commonly referred to as a drug misadventure?

   A. drug-drug interaction
   B. medication error
   C. adverse drug reaction
   D. all of the above

18. Most IV piggybacks contain fluid between 50 and:

   A. 100 mL
   B. 250 mL
   C. 500 mL
   D. 1000 mL

19. The patient profile is updated when:

   A. new medications are ordered and then expire
   B. new medications are delivered to the pharmacy
   C. new medications are ordered and previous orders are changed or discontinued
   D. the patient is discharged from the hospital

20. According to the ASHP Guidelines on Quality Assurance, sterile products that are stored at room temperature must be administered completely within:

   A. 12 hours
   B. 28 hours
   C. 48 hours
   D. 72 hours

21. Regular audits of personnel, equipment, facilities, policies, and procedure can help to:

   A. recognize the patient's need
   B. identify the cost of services
   C. identify problem areas
   D. all of the above

22. Computerized perpetual inventory systems are now in use to indicate. When medications should be:

   A. reordered
   B. stored
   C. returned
   D. sold

23. Which of the following is the most common type of sterile irrigation?

    A. surgical antibiotic solution
    B. antibiotic solution for the ear
    C. saline solution for the eye
    D. antibiotic solution for the urinary bladder

24. Clusters of bacteria growing in colonies are referred to as:

    A. diplococci
    B. streptococci
    C. staphylococci
    D. *E. coli*

25. The slanted part of a needle, at the tip of the shaft, is referred to as:

    A. the hub
    B. the shaft
    C. the bevel
    D. the gauge

26. Which of the following intravenous tubing is known as a "piggyback set"?

    A. primary
    B. secondary
    C. extension
    D. none of the above

27. Ophthalmics are sterile preparations intended for direct administration into the:

    A. retina
    B. iris
    C. pupil
    D. conjunctiva

28. Dark bags are used to keep medications away from direct light; they are tinted which of the following colors?

    A. brown
    B. green
    C. amber
    D. black

29. Which of the following are considered "durable medical goods"?

    A. IV poles
    B. infusion pumps
    C. wheelchairs
    D. containers

30. Primary IV tubing sets are sometimes called:

    A. vented tubing
    B. extension sets
    C. administration sets
    D. none of the above

31. Which of the following statements is true regarding the expiration date of drugs?

   A. Patients must be instructed to use their medications within 4 weeks after their expiration dates.
   B. Patients should never use their medications past their expiration dates.
   C. Patients are allowed to take certain medications within 6 months after their expiration dates.
   D. all of the above

32. Which of the following is used for computerized ordering systems?

   A. numeric identifiers
   B. national drug codes
   C. bar codes
   D. both A and C

33. Total parenteral nutrition is usually infused over a period of:

   A. 1 to 2 hours
   B. 4 to 6 hours
   C. 10 to 12 hours
   D. 48 to 72 hours

34. The pharmacy technician must use the appropriate form when returning defective items and fill in all of the following information, except the:

   A. original purchase order number
   B. quantity
   C. DEA number
   D. item number

35. Pharmacies must conduct a physical count of all controlled substances at least every:

   A. year
   B. 2 years
   C. 3 years
   D. 5 years

36. All of the following factors affect parenteral products, except:

   A. agent names
   B. pharmacokinetics
   C. solubility
   D. compatibility

37. Which of the following is an advantage of the unit-dose system?

   A. It is cheaper.
   B. It increases cross-contamination.
   C. It decreases the chance of medication errors.
   D. It increases the effect of medications.

38. The physical removal of debris, blood, and body fluids from instruments is referred to as:

   A. cleaning
   B. disinfection
   C. sterilization
   D. all of the above

39. Which of the following statements is true?

   A. Legend drugs must be dispensed only by a licensed pharmacist.
   B. Legend drugs may be dispensed by a licensed pharmacy technician.
   C. Pharmacy technicians can handle floor orders.
   D. both A and C

40. Which of the following is not a disadvantage of parenteral administration?

   A. local irritation
   B. difficulty in correcting errors
   C. risk of hepatic and renal toxicity
   D. pain

41. HEPA filters need to be certified every 6 months unless they become:

   A. dry
   B. wet
   C. dusted
   D. all of the above

42. Yeast infections may be caused by:

   A. bacteria
   B. fungi
   C. viruses
   D. protozoa

43. A pharmacy's inventory turnover rate indicates which of the following?

   A. how many times in a week that the inventory has been used or replaced
   B. how many times in a month that the inventory has been used or replaced
   C. how many times in a year that the inventory has been used or replaced
   D. none of the above

44. The clean room is designed to minimize the risk of infection from airborne pathogens via the use of:

   A. disposable syringes
   B. microscopes
   C. autoclaves
   D. laminar-airflow systems

45. Which of the following is a true statement?

   A. Those who deal with sterile compounding are required to have in-depth training and appropriate academic education.
   B. Those who deal with sterile compounding are required to be licensed pharmacists.
   C. Those who deal with sterile compounding are required to be certified pharmacy technicians.
   D. all of the above

46. Which of the following sources of nutrition should always be added into a total parenteral solution bag?

   A. sugars
   B. proteins
   C. lipids
   D. vitamins

47. All of the following are advantages of Viaflex bags, except:

    A. they are very resistant to breakage
    B. they are easy to handle
    C. they are inexpensive
    D. they are available in 50 to 100 mL sizes

48. Storage shelves in the clean room should be emptied completely every _____, and then cleaned and sanitized:

    A. day
    B. week
    C. 2 weeks
    D. month

49. Auxiliary labels help in which of the following?

    A. correct storage
    B. correct dosage
    C. correct price of medication
    D. all of the above

50. Which of the following is not required to be double-checked during the quality assurance process?

    A. the expiration date of the bulk product being used
    B. calculations used for reconstituting drug products
    C. the drug and dosage form being repackaged
    D. both A and B

51. Hoods must be thoroughly cleaned about every:

    A. hour
    B. 3 hours
    C. 5 hours
    D. 8 hours

52. Which of the following agencies or organizations ensure that safe and effective drugs are available in the United States?

    A. the Joint Commission
    B. the Center for Disease Control and Prevention
    C. the Center for Drug Evaluation and Research
    D. all of the above

53. Which of the following decrease the risk of contamination when a pharmacy technician prepares an IV admixture?

    A. ultraviolet lighting
    B. foot pedal sinks
    C. humidifiers
    D. laminar-airflow hoods

54. Which of the following is the mission of the American Medical Association?

    A. to prevent medication errors
    B. to promote the art and science of medicine for the betterment of public health
    C. to encourage manufacturers to do research for the treatment of rare diseases
    D. none of the above

55. How many pairs of latex gloves should be worn when preparing IV admixtures?

    A. 1
    B. 2
    C. 3
    D. none

56. Which of the following is the slanted part at the tip of the needle shaft?

    A. bevel
    B. hub
    C. tip
    D. none of the above

57. Electronic devices for infusion are mechanisms powdered by which of the following?

    A. batteries
    B. electricity
    C. water pressure
    D. both A and B

58. Most sharps containers are of which color?

    A. blue
    B. yellow
    C. red
    D. black

59. Continuous infusion is used for which of the following?

    A. when constant plasma drug concentration is required
    B. when highly diluted drugs are needed
    C. when large amounts of electrolytes and fluids must be replaced in the body
    D. all of the above

60. A drug's shelf life is based on which of the following factors?

    A. its stability
    B. the length of time it can be kept in stock before its contents become altered
    C. an expiration date
    D. all of the above

Matching

    1. _____ The process of preventing growth of microbes

    2. _____ Bypassing the skin and gastrointestinal tract (injected)

    3. _____ Causes molds and yeasts

    4. _____ A company that sells drugs

    5. _____ The smallest of microorganisms

    6. _____ A flexible rubber dome-shaped cup

    7. _____ Examination conducted to assure effectiveness and correctness

    8. _____ A carrier of an infectious agent

9. _____ A device used to separate certain elements or particles from a solution

10. _____ A system of tracking of drugs received by and sold in the pharmacy

    A. Perpetual inventory
    B. Diaphragm
    C. Audit
    D. Vendor
    E. Parenteral
    F. Filter
    G. Vector
    H. Virus
    I. Protozoa
    J. Asepsis
    K. Fungi

Fill in the Blank

1. A direct purchase is one that is made directly from the _____ by the pharmacy.

2. Controlled substances require detailed record keeping because they have high _____.

3. Chemotherapy drugs are usually kept in their own secured area of the pharmacy due to their _____.

4. Containing unwanted substances or organisms is referred to as _____.

5. The pharmacy technician must use appropriate _____ when returning goods.

6. Horizontal laminar-airflow hoods are used for preparation of parenteral medications and sterile product mixtures, and not for _____ agents.

7. Quality improvement strives continued quality over _____.

8. IV mixtures are prepared inside _____ within the hospital pharmacy to minimize risk of _____.

9. Bacteria that are arranged in _____ are known as diplococci.

10. Legend drugs must be dispensed by a _____ pharmacist.

11. Personnel are required to wear gowns, caps, gloves, and masks when dealing with _____.

12. Positively pressured flowing air that bathes a work area is referred to as _____.

13. Since many IV medications have a short _____ life, their admixtures are prepared when needed by a patient.

14. During the preparation, compounding, and administration of parenteral medications, the parts of a syringe must remain _____.

15. Level 1 in the ASHP Guideline includes products to be stored at room temperature and administered completely with _____ after being prepared.

16. The controlled flow of an intravenous medication into a patient is called _____.

17. Multi-dose vials are used for injectables that are not available in _____ doses.

18. USP <797> lists all necessary _____ processes.

19. To disinfect countertop surfaces in the laboratory, the least expensive and most readily available chemical is ordinary _____.

20. Most ampoules have a constriction in the stem that is marked with a _____.

21. The most important health procedure that can be performed to prevent the spread of microbes is _____.

22. Cardboard items should never be placed in _____ because they contain free-floating particles.

23. Autoclaves use steam under pressure to obtain temperatures of approximately _____ degrees Fahrenheit.

24. The American Medical Association publishes the _____ *of the American Medical Association* as well as many other documents.

25. Excessive air forced into a _____ can aerosolize the contents into the air or even burst the vial.

26. Primary IV tubing is usually 60 inches or longer, and can be used with IV _____ or by itself for gravity _____.

27. Total nutrient admixtures are designed to provide all _____ to a patient in a single delivery system.

28. Garments are sometimes referred to as _____.

29. Types of IV medications include IV push, used for rapid infusion, and _____ devices, which regulate the infusion of IV substances.

30. Port adapters are "male" adapters that are attached to the IV _____ post of an IV bag.

True or False

1. _____ Parenteral products can be compounded into small-volume or large-volume IV bags.

2. _____ Ophthalmics are sterile preparations intended for direct administration into the retina.

3. _____ Rapid direct injection is also known as "bolus."

4. _____ The process of inhibiting growth of microorganisms is called "microbiology."

5. _____ Most of the furniture found in a clean room is made of wood, which can be easily cleaned with wood alcohol.

6. _____ The skin and hair of pharmacy technicians are reservoirs for bacteria.

7. _____ Popular large-volume parenterals include 0.9% sodium chloride, and 5% dextrose in water.

8. _____ Most sterile preparation programs use special computer software at dedicated terminals in specific areas away from the sterile preparation area.

9. _____ For sterile compounding of pharmaceutical agents, there are specialized work areas where air quality, humidity, and temperature are highly regulated.

10. _____ For aseptic technique, the hands, wrists, and arms up to the elbow should be washed with cold water and antimicrobial soap for 3 to 5 minutes.

11. _____ Ophthalmic drops contain filtered elements that are safe to use.

12. _____ The drug inventory in a pharmaceutical compounding pharmacy is generally different from that of other types of pharmacies.

13. _____ Both prescription medications and OTC products must be routinely checked for reaching their expiration dates.

14. _____ The manufacturer offers the highest price and requires a maximum quantity order.

15. _____ An NDC number uniquely identifies each drug product and indicates the manufacturer's name, the drug's name, its strength, its dosage form, and the package size of the drug product.

16. _____ An invoice is a listing of items in a shipment without the prices shown.

17. _____ Storage of drugs must be handled by following the FDA recommendation for temperature, light exposure, humidity, and other factors.

18. _____ Quality assurance process checkpoints may include double-checking of the drug and dosage form being repackaged.

19. _____ USP Chapter <797> is the first enforceable set of standards defining many quality control areas.

20. _____ Horizontal airflow hoods are used for chemotherapeutic agents.

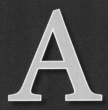

APPENDIX A

Sample MSDS

Material Safety Data Sheet

Version 1.8
Revision Date 08/22/2004

MSDS Number 300000000110
Print Date 09/21/2008

1. PRODUCT AND COMPANY IDENTIFICATION

Product name   : Oxygen
Chemical formula   : O_2
Synonyms   : Oxygen, Oxygen Gas, Gaseous Oxygen, GOX
Product use description   : General Industrial
Company   : Air Products and Chemicals, Inc
                                       7201 Hamilton Blvd.
                                       Allentown, PA 18195-1501
Telephone   : 1-800-345-3148 Chemicals
                                       1-800-752-1597 Gases and Electronic Chemicals
Emergency telephone number   : 800-523-9374 USA
                                       01-610-481-7711 International

2. COMPOSITION/INFORMATION ON INGREDIENTS

Components	CAS Number	Concentration (Volume)
Oxygen	7782-44-7	100%

Concentration is nominal. For the exact product composition, please refer to Air Products technical specifications.

Material Safety Data Sheet

Version 1.8
Revision Date 08/22/2004

MSDS Number 300000000110
Print Date 09/21/2008

3. HAZARDS IDENTIFICATION

Emergency Overview

High pressure, oxidizing gas.
Vigorously accelerates combustion.
Keep oil, grease, and combustibles away.
May react violently with combustible materials.

Potential Health Effects

Inhalation	: Breathing 75% or more oxygen at atmospheric pressure for more than a few hours may cause nasal stuffiness, cough, sore throat, chest pain and breathing difficulty. Breathing pure oxygen under pressure may cause lung damage and also central nervous system effects.
Eye contact	: No adverse effect.
Skin contact	: No adverse effect.
Ingestion	: Ingestion is not considered a potential route of exposure.

Exposure Guidelines

Primary Routes of Entry	: Inhalation
Target Organs	: None known.

Aggravated Medical Condition

If oxygen is administered to persons with chronic obstructive pulmonary disease, raising the oxygen concentration in the blood depresses their breathing and raises their retained carbon dioxide to a dangerous level.

4. FIRST AID MEASURES

General advice	: Remove victim to uncontaminated area wearing self-contained breathing apparatus. Keep victim warm and rested. Call a doctor. Apply artificial respiration if breathing stopped.
Eye contact	: Seek medical advice.
Skin contact	: Wash with water and soap as a precaution.
Ingestion	: Ingestion is not considered a potential route of exposure.
Inhalation	: Consult a physician after significant exposure. Move to fresh air. If breathing has stopped or is labored, give assisted respirations. Supplemental oxygen may be indicated. If the heart has stopped, trained personnel should begin cardiopulmonary resuscitation immediately.

Material Safety Data Sheet

Version 1.8
Revision Date 08/22/2004

MSDS Number 300000000110
Print Date 09/21/2008

5. FIRE-FIGHTING MEAURES

Suitable extinguishing media	: All known extinguishing media can be used.
Special hazards	: Most cylinders are designed to vent contents when exposed to elevated temperatures.
Further information	: Some materials that are noncombustible in air will burn in the presence of an oxygen enriched atmosphere (greater than 23%). Fire resistant clothing may burn and offer no protection in oxygen rich atmospheres.

6. ACCIDENTAL RELEASE MEASURES

Personal precautions	: Clothing exposed to high concentrations may retain oxygen 30 minutes or longer and become a potential fire hazard. Stay away from ignition sources. Evacuate personnel to safe areas. Wear self-contained breathing apparatus when entering area unless atmosphere is proved to be safe. Ventilate the area.
Environmental precautions	: Do not discharge into any place where its accumulation could be dangerous. Prevent further leakage or spillage if safe to do so.
Methods for cleaning up	: Ventilate the area.
Additional advice	: If possible, stop flow of product. Increase ventilation to the release area and monitor concentrations. If leak is from cylinder valve, call the Air Products emergency telephone number. If the leak is in the user's system, close the cylinder valve, safely vent the pressure, and purge with an inert gas before attempting repairs.

7. HANDLING AND STORAGE

Handling

All gauges, valves, regulators, piping and equipment to be used in oxygen service must be cleaned for oxygen service. Oxygen is not to be used as a substitute for compressed air. Never use an oxygen jet for cleaning purposes of any sort, especially clothing, as it increases the likelihood of an engulfing fire. Only experienced and properly instructed persons should handle compressed gases. Protect cylinders from physical damage; do not drag, roll, slide, or drop. Do not allow storage area temperature to exceed 50°C (122°F). Before using the product, determine its identity by reading the label. Know and understand the properties and hazards of the product before use. When doubt exists as to the correct handling procedure for a particular gas, contact the supplier. Do not remove or deface labels provided by the supplier for the identification of the cylinder contents. When moving cylinders, even for short distances, use a cart (trolley, hand truck, etc.) designed to transport cylinders. Leave valve protection caps in place until the container has been secured against either a wall or bench or placed in a container stand and is ready for use. Use an adjustable strap wrench to remove over-tight or rusted caps. Before connecting the container, check the complete gas system for suitability, particularly for pressure rating and materials. Before connecting the container for use, ensure that back feed from the system into the container is prevented. Ensure the complete gas system is compatible for pressure rating and materials of construction. Ensure the complete gas system has been checked for leaks before use. Employ suitable pressure regulating devices on all

Material Safety Data Sheet

Version 1.8
Revision Date 08/22/2004

MSDS Number 300000000110
Print Date 09/21/2008

---

containers when the gas is being emitted to systems with lower pressure rating than that of the container. Never insert an object (e.g., wrench, screwdriver, pry bar, etc.) into valve cap openings. Doing so may damage valve, causing a leak to occur. If user experiences any difficulty operating cylinder valve discontinue use and contact supplier. Close container valve after each use and when empty, even if still connected to equipment. Never attempt to repair or modify container valves or safety relief devices. Damaged valves should be reported immediately to the supplier. Do not use containers as rollers or supports or for any other purpose than to contain the gas as supplied. Never strike an arc on a compressed gas cylinder or make a cylinder a part of an electrical circuit. Do not smoke while handling product or cylinders. Never recompress a gas or a gas mixture without first consulting the supplier. Never attempt to transfer gases from one cylinder/container to another. Always use backflow protective device in piping. When returning cylinder install valve outlet cap or plug leak tight. Never permit oil, grease, or other readily combustible substances to come into contact with valves or containers containing oxygen or other oxidants. Do not use rapidly opening valves (e.g., ball valves). Open valve slowly to avoid pressure shock. Never pressurize the entire system at once. Use only with equipment cleaned for oxygen service and rated for cylinder pressure. Never use direct flame or electrical heating devices to raise the pressure of a container. Containers should not be subjected to temperatures above 50ºC (122ºF). Prolonged periods of cold temperature below –30ºC (–20ºF) should be avoided.

Storage

Containers should be stored in a purpose build compound which should be well ventilated, preferably in the open air. Full containers should be stored so that oldest stock is used first. Stored containers should be periodically checked for general condition and leakage. Observe all regulations and local requirements regarding storage of containers. Protect containers stored in the open against rusting and extremes of weather. Containers should not be stored in conditions likely to encourage corrosion. Containers should be stored in the vertical position and properly secured to prevent toppling. The container valves should be tightly closed and where appropriate valve cutlets should be capped or plugged. Container valve guards or caps should be in place. Keep containers tightly closed in a cool, well-ventilated place. Store containers in location free from fire risk and away from sources of heat and ignition. Full and empty cylinders should be segregated. Do not allow storage temperature to exceed 50ºC (122ºF). Display "No Smoking or Open Flames" signs in the storage areas. Return empty containers in a timely manner. Flammable storage areas should be separated from oxygen and other oxidizers by a minimum distance of 20 ft. (6.1 m.) or by a barrier of non-combustible material at least 5 ft. (1.5 m.) high, having a fire resistance rating of at least ½ hour.

Technical measures/Precautions

Containers should be segregated in the storage area according to the various categories (e.g., flammable, toxic, etc.) and in accordance with local regulations.

---

8. EXPOSURE CONTROLS / PERSONAL PROTECTION

Personal protective equipment

Respiratory protection	: Users of breathing apparatus must be trained.
Hand protection	: Sturdy work gloves are recommended for handling cylinders. The breakthrough time of the selected glove(s) must be greater than the intended use period.
Eye protection	: Safety glasses recommended when handling cylinders.
Skin and body protection	: Safety shoes are recommended when handling cylinders.

Material Safety Data Sheet
Version 1.8
Revision Date 08/22/2004

MSDS Number 300000000110
Print Date 09/21/2008

Special instructions for protection and hygiene	: Ensure adequate ventilation, especially in confined areas. Gloves must be clean and free of oil and grease.

9. PHYSICAL AND CHEMICAL PROPERTIES

Form	: Compressed gas.
Color	: Colorless gas.
Odor	: No odor warning properties.
Molecular weight	: 32 g/mol
Relative vapor density	: 1.1 (air = 1)
Relative density	: 1.1 (water = 1)
Density	: 0.081 lb/ft^3 (0.0013 g/cm^3) at 70°F (21°C) Note: (as vapor)
Specific volume	: 12.08 ft^3/lb (0.7540 m^3/kg) at 70°F (21°C)
Boiling point/range	: –297°F (–183°C)
Critical temperature	: –180°F (–118°C)
Melting point/range	: –362°F (–219°C)
Water solubility	: 0.039 g/l

10. STABILITY AND REACTIVITY

Stability	: Stable under normal conditions.
Materials to avoid	: Flammable materials. Organic materials. Avoid oil, grease, and all other combustible materials.

11. TOXICOLOGICAL INFORMATION

Acute Health Hazard

Ingestion	: No data is available on the product itself.
Inhalation	: No data is available on the product itself.
Skin	: No data is available on the product itself.

Chronic Health Hazard

Premature infants exposed to high concentrations may suffer delayed retinal damage that can progress to retinal detachment and blindness. Retinal damage may also occur in adults exposed to 100% oxygen for extended periods (24 to 48 hr). At two or more atmospheres central nervous system (CNS) toxicity occurs. Symptoms include nausea, vomiting, dizziness or vertigo, muscle twitching, vision changes, and loss of consciousness and generalized seizures. At three atmospheres, CNS toxicity occurs in less than two hours and six atmospheres in only a few minutes.

Material Safety Data Sheet

Version 1.8
Revision Date 08/22/2004

MSDS Number 300000000110
Print Date 09/21/2008

12. ECOLOGICAL INFORMATION

Ecotoxicity effects

Aquatic toxicity	: No data is available on the product itself.
Toxicity to other organisms	: No data available.

Persistence and degradability

Mobility	: No data available.
Bioaccumulation	: No data is available on the product itself.

Further information

No ecological damage caused by this product.

13. DISPOSAL CONSIDERATIONS

Waste from residues / unused products	: Return unused product in original cylinder to supplier. Contact supplier if guidance is required.
Contaminated packaging	: Return cylinder to supplier.

14. TRANSPORT INFORMATION

CFR

Proper shipping name	: Oxygen, compressed
Class	: 2.2 (5.1)
UN/ID No.	: UN1072

IATA

Proper shipping name	: Oxygen, compressed
Class	: 2.2 (5.1)
UN/ID No.	: UN1072

IMDG

Proper shipping name	: Oxygen, compressed
Class	: 2.2 (5.1)
UN/ID No.	: UN1072

CTC

Proper shipping name	: Oxygen, compressed
Class	: 2.2 (5.1)
UN/ID No.	: UN1072

Material Safety Data Sheet

Version 1.8
Revision Date 08/22/2004

Further Information

Avoid transport on vehicles where the load space is not separated from the driver's compartment. Ensure vehicle driver is aware of the potential hazards of the load and knows what to do in the event of an accident or an emergency.

15. REGULATOR / INFORMATION

OSHA Hazard Communication Standard (29 CFR 1910.1200) Hazard Class(es)
Oxidizer. Compressed Gas.

Country	Regulatory list	Notification
USA	TSCA	Included on Inventory.
EU	EINECS	Included on Inventory.
Canada	DSL	Included on Inventory.
Australia	AICS	Included on Inventory.
South Korea	ECL	Included on Inventory.
China	SEPA	Included on Inventory.
Philippines	PICCS	Included on Inventory.
Japan	ENCS	Included on Inventory.

EPA SARA Title III Section 312 (40 CFR 370) Hazard Classification:
Fire Hazard. Sudden Release of Pressure Hazard.

US. California Safe Drinking Water & Toxic Enforcement Act (Proposition 65)
This product does not contain any chemicals known to State of California to cause cancer, birth defects, or any other harm.

16. OTHER INFORMATION

NFPA Rating

Health	: 0
Fire	: 0
Instability	: 0
Special	: OX

HMIS Rating

Health	: 0
Flammability	: 0
Physical hazard	: 3
Prepared by	: Air Products and Chemicals, Inc. Global EH&S Product Safety Department

For additional information, please visit our Product Stewardship web site at
http//www.airproducts.com/productstewardship/

Reprinted with permission of Air Products and Chemicals Inc.

B Examples of Compounding Formulas

Note: These are actual compounding formulas from a variety of sources. Each is unique to the type of medication being prepared. There is no single standard for compounding formulas.

1. Allopurinol suspension

Allopurinol tablets	qs
Citric acid	250 mg
Methylcellulose 1%	50 mL
Cherry-flavored syrup	20 mL
Water	Up to 100 mL

Use 50 mL of methylcellulose 1% solution or 0.5 g per 100 mL. Reduce the amount if the final mixture is too viscous. The mixture will expire in 30 days. It must be refrigerated and protected from light. It must be shaken well before use.

2. Cefazolin eye drops

Cefazolin	1 g (vial)
Liquifilm tears or Tears Naturale®	7 cc
PF saline	2.5 cc

Add 2.5 cc of PF saline to 1 g (vial) of cefazolin. Add the mixture to 7 cc of Liquifilm tears or Tears Naturale. The final concentration will be 100 mg/cc.

3. Cocaine 5% – for topical use [for hospital pharmacy]

Cocaine 5%	5 g (bottle)
Methylene blue (tinting agent)	0.5 cc
Sterile water for irrigation, qs	Up to 100 mL

Mix cocaine with sterile water up to the required amount. Add methylene blue to tint. Transfer 10 mL of mixture into a 1 oz amber bottle; this is the total dosage allowed for each topical use. Repeat until all of the mixture has been bottled accordingly. Bottles must be labeled: "Cocaine Solution 5% – Topical Use Only – 10 mL." The expiration date is 3 months from the date of mixture. Each bottle must be signed out of the hospital pharmacy individually for use.

4. Gastrointestinal cocktail

Donnatal® Elixir	100 mL
Mylanta II	300 mL
Viscous xylocaine	50 mL

Combine the ingredients using an alcohol cabinet—the mixture is light-sensitive and must be bottled accordingly. The final amount will total 450 mL, of which the usual dose is 45 mL. It must be shaken well before use.

5. Genamicin eye drops (fortified)

Garamycin® eye drops 3 mg/cc	5 cc
Garamycin injection 80 mg/2cc	2 cc

Add 2 cc of Garamycin injection to a 5 cc bottle of Garamycin eye drops.

Total volume 95 mg = 13.57 mg/cc

6. Granisetron hydrochloride solution

Cherry syrup	120 mL
Granisetron (1 mg tablet)	24 tablets
Sterile water for irrigation	60 mL

Grind tablets to a fine powder using a mortar and pestle. Levigate with sterile water until a paste is formed, adding the water in increasing amounts while mixing. Transfer to a graduated cylinder, making sure to rinse the mortar and pestle with the base solution, pouring this into the graduated cylinder as well. Add the remainder of the base solution until the total volume is reached. Transfer the mixture into the appropriately sized amber-colored bottle. Shake well to mix. Store at room temperature or in a refrigerator. It must be shaken well before use. The mixture expires within 14 days.

7. Hydrocortisone 10%/ultrasound lotion

Ethyl alcohol 50%	50 mL
Hydrocortisone	25 g
Ultrasound lotion	255 mL

Place hydrocortisone in a mortar. Add ethyl alcohol, grinding and mixing until smooth. While stirring with the pestle, add ultrasound lotion slowly until the lotion is smooth. Transfer the mixture into an appropriate container (1 oz bottle). The mixture expires in 6 months. It must be shaken well before use.

8. Lidocaine – epinephrine – tetracaine gel

K-Y® Jelly	22.5 mL
Lidocaine 20%	10 mL
Racemic epinephrine 2.25%	5 mL
Sodium metabisulfite	31.5 mg
Tetracaine 2%	12.5 mL

The final preparation provides approximately 50 mL of gel. Divide into 9 or 10 single-use containers holding 5 mL each. Store in refrigerator. The gel expires within 5 months.

9. Phenoxybenzamine solution 2 mg/mL

Citric acid powder	45 mg
Phenoxybenzamine 10 mg capsule	6 capsules
Propylene glycol	0.3 mL
Sterile water for irrigation	30 mL

Empty the contents of the capsules into a mortar and grind to a fine powder. Add citric acid and propylene glycol. Levigate with a small amount of the base solution to form a paste, adding base solution while mixing thoroughly. Transfer to a graduated cylinder. Rinse the mortar and pestle with base solution and pour it into a graduated cylinder to achieve the total volume required. Transfer the solution into an appropriately sized amber-colored bottle. Shake well to mix. Store in a refrigerator. Shake well before use. The solution expires in 7 days.

10. Pronestyl oral suspension (500 mg per 10 mL)

Glycerin	3 to 5 cc
Pronestyl® (500 mg capsules)	12 capsules
Sorbitol (optional)	as needed
Sterile water, qs	120 cc

Empty the contents of Pronestyl capsules into a mortar. Add glycerin to make a smooth preparation. Add sterile water to required amount while mixing. Add sorbitol if required for better flavor. Store at room temperature; do not refrigerate. It must be shaken well before use.

C Sample Physician Orders for Sterile Compounding

1. Valproate Sodium [Depacon EQ] — 750 mg/7.5 mL

   Sodium Chloride 0.9% — 100 mL
   Freq: Q4H — RT: IV
   Infuse over 30 Minutes
   Expires in 48 Hours

2. **STOP** Caution: Pediatric Patient

Dextrose 50%	36 mL
Aminosyn-PF 10%	56.43 mL
Cysteine HCL	4.51 mL
Sodium Phosphate	0.35 mL
Sodium Chloride	0.35 mL
Sodium Acetate	0 mL
Potassium Chloride	0 mL
Potassium Acetate	1.41 mL
Potassium Phosphate	0 mL
Magnesium Sulfate	0.07 mL
Calcium Gluconate	5.64 mL
Heparin Flush (PF)	0 mL

3. **STOP** Caution: Pediatric Patient

   Trace Metals Pediatric — 0.45 mL
   Pediatric Multivitamins — 4.5 mL
   Water — 70.28 mL
   Tot Vol = 180 mL Dex Conc = 10%
   Rate: 5 mL/hr — RT: IV
   Expires in 36 Hours

4. Sodium Chloride 0.9% — 100 mL

   Pantoprazole Sod — 80 mg
   Sesquihydrate
   Rate: 10 mL/hr — RT: IV
   Expires in 48 Hours

5. Penicillin G Potassium — 2.5 mu/5 mL
   [Penicillin G Potassium]

   Dextrose 5% 5% — 100 mL
   2.5 mu = 2.5 Million Units PCN
   Q4H Until Delivery. Notify Rx
   Refrigerate
   Freq: Q4H — RT: IV
   Infuse over 30 Minutes
   Expires in 24 Hours

6. Tigecycline [Tygacil] — 50 mg

   Sodium Chloride 0.9% — 100 mL
   Keep Refrigerated
   At Room Temp Expires
   6 Hours after Preparation
   Freq: Q12H — RT: IV
   Infuse over 30 Minutes
   Expires in 24 Hours

7. Azithromycin [Zithromax EQ] — 500 mg

   Sodium Chloride 0.9% — 250 mL
   Stored in Refrigerator
   Freq: Q24H — RT: IV
   Infuse over 1 Hour
   Expires in 48 Hours

8. Vancomycin HCL
   [Vancomycin HCL] — 1,500 mg

   Dextrose 5% in Water (D5W) — 250 mL
   Freq: Q12H — RT: IV
   Infuse over 90 Minutes
   Expires in 48 Hours

9. NACL 0.45%-KCL 20 meq/L — 1,000 mL

   Thiamine Hcl — 100 mg
   Folic Acid — 1 mg
   Rate: 100 mL/hr — RT: IV
   Expires in 48 Hours

10. Imipenem-Cilastatin
    [Primaxin IV]   500 mg

    Sodium Chloride 0.9%   100 mL
    Freq: Q8H   RT: IV
    Infuse over 60 Minutes
    Expires in 24 Hours

11. **STOP**   Caution: Pediatric Patient

    Ampicillin Sodium/NS   150 mg/6 mL
    [Ampicillin Sodium/Saline]
    Stored in Refrigerator
    200 mg/Kg/Day @ 3 Kg
    ** Note Volume **
    *** Dispense in 20 mL Syringe or
    Small IV Bag Depending
    on Volume ***
    **** Pediatric Dose ****
    Stable for 8 Hours after
        Preparation
    Freq: Q6H   RT: IV
    Infuse over 30 Minutes
    Expires in 24 Hours

12. Levetiracetam [Keppra]   1,500 mg/15 mL

    Sodium Chloride 0.9%   100 mL
    Freq: Q12H   RT: IV
    Infuse over 30 Minutes
    Expires in 48 Hours

13. Vancomycin HCL
    [Vancomycin HCL]   2,000 mg

    Dextrose 5% in Water (D5W)   500 mL
    Freq: Q24H   RT: IV
    Infuse over 2 Hours
    Expires in 48 Hours

14. Clindamycin Phosphate in D5W   140 mg/7.78 mL
    [Cleocin in D5W]

    Pat Wt = 14 Kg × 10 mg/Kg =
        140 mg Dose
    ** Note Volume **
    *** Dispense in 20 mL Syringe or
    Small IV Bag Depending
    on Volume ***
    **** Pediatric Dose ****
    Freq: Q6H   RT: IV
    Infuse over 30 Minutes
    Expires in 48 Hours

15. Methocarbamol [Robaxin]   500 mg/5 mL

    Sodium Chloride 0.9%   100 mL
    Do Not Refrigerate!!
    Freq: Q6H   RT: IV

    Infuse over 60 Minutes
    Expires in 48 Hours

16. Meropenem [Merrem]   1 G

    Sodium Chloride 0.9%   100 mL
    Expires after 4 Hours at Room
        Temp or
    24 Hours if Refrigerated.
    Freq: Q8H   RT: IV
    Infuse over 30 Minutes
    Expires in 48 Hours

17. Vancomycin HCL
    [Vancomycin HCL]   750 mg

    Dextrose 5% In Water (D5W)   250 mL
    Freq: Q12H   RT: IV
    Infuse over 60 Minutes
    Expires in 48 Hours

18. Ertapenem Sodium [Invanz]   1 g

    Sodium Chloride 0.9%   50 mL
    Expires 6 Hours after Preparation if
    Kept at Room Temp
    Stable for 24 Hours under
        Refrigeration
    Freq: Q24H   RT: IV
    Infuse over 30 Minutes
    Expires in 48 Hours

19. Ampicillin-Sulbactam [Unasyn]   1.5 gm

    Sodium Chloride 0.9%   50 mL
    Stored in Refrigerator
    Freq: Q8H   RT: IV
    Infuse over 30 Minutes
    Expires in 48 Hours

20. Cefoxitin Sodium [Mefoxin EQ]   1 g

    Dextrose 5%   50 mL
    Freq: Q6H   RT: IV
    Infuse over 30 Minutes
    Expires in 48 Hours

21. Cefepime HCL [Maxipime EQ]   2 gram

    Sodium Chloride 0.9%   100 mL
    Freq: Q8H   RT: IV
    Infuse over 1 Hour
    Expires in 48 Hours

22. Dextrose 50%   500 mL

    Amino Acids 8.5%   500 mL
    Sodium   37 meq
    Potassium   45 meq
    Calcium   5 meq
    Magnesium   5 meq
    Chloride   94 meq
    Phosphate   9 mmoles

Acetate   47 meq

Central Line Tpn

Rate: 90 mL/hr   RT: IV

Expires in 48 Hours

23. Dextrose 50%   500 mL

    Amino Acids 10%   500 mL
    Sodium   38 meq
    Potassium   27 meq
    Calcium   5 meq
    Magnesium   5 meq
    Chloride   75 meq
    Phosphate   6 mmo
    Acetate   52 meq
    Multiple Vitamins   10 mL
    Trace Elements   1 mL
    Central Line TPN-Modified Protein

Rate: 55 mL/hr   RT: IV

Expires in 48 Hours

24. Dextrose 50%   500 mL

    Amino Acids 8.5%   500 mL
    Sodium   38 meq
    Potassium   27 meq
    Calcium   5 meq
    Magnesium   5 meq
    Chloride   72 meq
    Phosphate   6 mmo
    Acetate   47 meq
    Multiple Vitamins   10 mL
    Trace Elements   1 mL
    Central Line TPN
    Rate: 60 mL/hr   RT: IV
    Expires in 48 Hours

D Dosage Calculations

Using Ratios and Proportions to Calculate Dosages

1. Ratios may be written as 3 : 4, meaning that there are 3 parts of drug #1 to 4 parts of solution or solvent. *Ratios* express the relationship between two or more quantities. Ratios are usually shown as fractions in drug calculations, as follows:

$$\frac{3 \text{ parts of drug \#1}}{4 \text{ parts of a solution}} = \frac{3}{4}$$

Proportions show the relationship between two ratios:

$$\frac{\text{Dose on hand}}{\text{Quantity on hand}} = \frac{\text{Desired dose}}{\text{Desired quantity (X)}}$$

The same formula can be shown as follows, by using cross multiplication:

$$\text{Desired quantity (X)} = \frac{\text{Desired dose}}{\text{Dose on hand} \times \text{Quantity on hand}}$$

Question: If the dose on hand is 200 mg, the desired dose is 400 mg, and the quantity on hand is 10 mL, what is the desired quantity (X)?

$$\frac{\text{Dose on hand (200 mg)}}{\text{Quantity on hand (10 mL)}} = \frac{\text{Desired dose (400 mg)}}{\text{Desired quantity (X)}}$$

When cross multiplying, we find:

$$200 \times X = 10 \text{ mL} \times 400$$
$$200 \text{ X} = 4{,}000 \text{ mL}$$
$$X = 20 \text{ mL}$$

The dose to be administered is 20 mL.

2. The same proportion method can solve solid dosage calculations, as follows:

If the dose on hand is available as 5 mg tablets, and the desired dose is 25 mg/day, how many tablets should be administered each day?

$$\frac{\text{Dose on hand (5 mg)}}{1 \text{ tablet}} = \frac{\text{Desired dose (25 mg)}}{\text{Desired quantity (X)}}$$

By cross-multiplying, it is found that:

$$5 \text{ mg} \times X = 25 \text{ mg} \times 1 \text{ tablet}$$
$$5 \text{ X} = 25 \text{ mg}$$
$$X = 5 \text{ tablets/day}$$

Therefore, 5 tablets should be administered daily.

Dosage Calculations by Weight

Drug dosages are often expressed as milligrams per unit of body weight (usually kilograms rather than pounds), and are commonly used in depicting pediatric doses. An example of a recommended dose of a drug might be 1 mg/kg/24 hours. This information can be used to calculate the dose for a specific patient, or to check that prescribed doses are correct and not significantly under or over the required doses for that patient.

Caution must always be used in converting between pounds and kilograms. The formula that should be understood is as follows:

$$\text{Body weight} \times (\text{dose in mg/kg}) = X \text{ mg of drug}$$

Example: Chewable tablets for a 110-pound child are to be administered at the rate of 20 mg/kg/dose. How many tablets, if they are 500 mg each, should be administered to this patient for each dose?

First, convert the patient's weight to kilograms as follows:

$$1 \text{ kg} = 2.2 \text{ lbs}$$

$$\frac{1 \text{ kg}}{2.2 \text{ lbs}} = \frac{X \text{ kg}}{110 \text{ lbs}}$$

$$X = 50 \text{ kg}$$

Next, calculate the total daily dose as follows. For each kg of body weight, you should give 20 mg of the drug.

$$\frac{20 \text{ mg}}{1 \text{ kg}} = \frac{X \text{ mg}}{50 \text{ kg}}$$

$$X = 1,000 \text{ mg}$$

Finally, calculate the number of tablets needed to supply 1,000 mg per dose. Remember that the concentration of the tablets on hand is 500 mg per tablet.

$$\frac{500 \text{ mg}}{1 \text{ tablet}} = \frac{1,000 \text{ mg}}{X \text{ tablets}}$$

$$X = 2 \text{ tablets per dose}$$

Dosage Calculations by Body Surface Area

Using body surface area to calculate pediatric dosages is a very accurate method. Nomograms are charts that use patient weight and height to determine body surface area in square meters (m^2). This body surface area (BSA) is then placed into a ratio with the average adult's body surface area (1.73 m^2). The following formula is then used:

$$\text{Child's dose} = \frac{\text{Child's BSA in m}^2}{1.73 \text{ m}^2} \times \text{Adult dose}$$

Nomogram scales contain metric and avoirdupois values for height and weight, enabling body surface area to be determined in pounds and inches or kilograms and centimeters without needing to make conversions (see the illustration of the nomogram scale in Appendix E).

To determine BSA, a ruler or straightedge is recommended. After determining the patient's height and weight, place the ruler or straightedge on the nomogram and connect the two points on the height and weight scales that represent the patient's values. Where the ruler or straightedge crosses the center column (BSA), the corresponding reading

is the value of the BSA in square meters. Substitute the BSA value in the formula to calculate the dosage for this patient. If this child's BSA is 0.52 m^2, and the adult dosage of the required drug is 500 mg, use the following formula to determine the child's dose:

$$\text{Child's dose} = \frac{0.52 \text{ m}^2}{1.73 \text{ m}^2} \times \text{Adult dose (500 mg)}$$

$$= 0.3 \times 500 \text{ mg}$$

$$= 150 \text{ mg (child's dose)}$$

How to Calculate IV Infusion Rates

To calculate the flow rate using the ratio and proportion method, follow these steps:

1. Determine the number of milliliters the patient will receive per hour
2. Determine the number of milliliters the patient will receive per minute
3. Determine the number of drops per minute that will equal the number of milliliters calculated above. The IV set's drop rate must be considered. This is expressed as a ratio of drops per milliliter (gtt/mL).

Example: The prescriber orders 3,000 mL of dextrose 5% in water (D_5W) IV over 24 hours. If the IV set delivers 15 drops per milliliter, how many drops must be administered per minute?

First, calculate mL/hr.

$$\frac{3,000 \text{ mL}}{24 \text{ hrs}} = \frac{X \text{ mL}}{1 \text{ hr}}$$

$$X = 125 \text{ mL/hr or } 125 \text{ mL/60 min}$$

Next, calculate mL/min.

$$\frac{125 \text{ mL}}{60 \text{ min}} = \frac{X \text{ mL}}{1 \text{ min}}$$

$$X = 2 \text{ mL/min}$$

Finally, calculate gtt/min using the drop rate per minute of the IV set. (IV set drop rate = 15 drops/mL)

$$\frac{15 \text{ gtt}}{1 \text{ mL}} = \frac{X \text{ gtt}}{2 \text{ mL (amount needed/min)}}$$

$$X = 30 \text{ gtt/min}$$

Nomogram

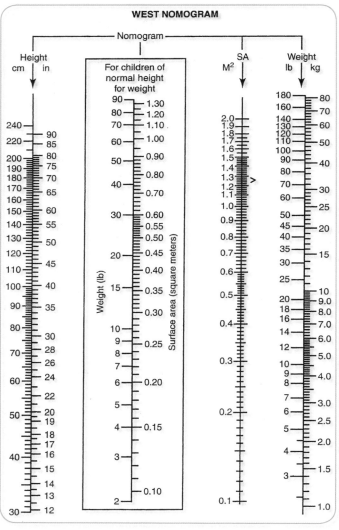

WEST NOMOGRAM

A nomogram is a chart that permits the estimation of body surface area (BSA) from the client's height and weight. Different charts are needed for children and adults (note children's box in diagram). To find the BSA for your client, record the client's weight on the weight scale by placing a dot at the appropriate spot. Do the same for the client's height on the height chart. Using a ruler, draw a straight line between the two dots. Where the line crosses the BSA graph, read the client's BSA. (From Behrman, R. E., Kleigman, R. M., & Arvin, A. M. (2000). *Nelson Textbook of Pediatrics* (16th ed.). Philadelphia: W. B. Saunders. Reprinted with permission.)

Answer Keys

Chapter 1

Multiple Choice

1. D	2. A	3. A	4. D	5. C	6. C
7. C	8. C	9. A	10. D	11. A	12. A

Fill in the Blank

1. jobs
2. OSHA
3. policy; procedures
4. reported
5. untargeted
6. ten
7. occupational
8. Labor
9. pathogenicity
10. rigid

Chapter 2

Multiple Choice

1. C	2. B	3. C	4. A	5. C
6. D	7. C	8. B	9. D	10. A

Matching

1. F	2. E	3. B	4. C	5. A	6. D

Fill in the Blank

1. rinsing
2. reference
3. C
4. biotransformation
5. buccal
6. distribution

Chapter 3

Multiple Choice

1. D	2. B	3. B	4. C	5. B
6. B	7. D	8. D	9. D	10. D

Matching

1. F	2. E	3. D	4. B	5. C	6. A

Fill in the Blank

1. radiopharmaceuticals
2. airflow hoods
3. piggybacks
4. compounding

Short Answer

1. The preparation, mixing, assembling, packaging, or labeling of a drug or device.

2. Daily intravenous medications, total parenteral nutrition (TPN) solutions, antibiotic piggybacks, IV additives, and pediatric dosage forms.

3. Hospital pharmacy compounding, ambulatory care compounding, nuclear pharmacy compounding.

4. Stability – properties of a substance that may be affected by temperature, light exposure, and specific container types.

   Equipment – clean air environments, electronic balances, ointment slabs, spatulas, mortars, pestles, glassware, and sterilization devices.

   Environment – a separate area that is clean, neat, well-lit, and quiet; aseptic conditions are usually required.

   Formulas – standards for compounding that ensure batch-to-batch consistency, documentable procedures, and proper preparation methods and ingredients.

Chemicals & supplies – proper vehicles (such as creams or ointments) as well as active ingredients (usually powders or chemicals) are required for effective compounding. Proper dispensing containers that will not compromise the effectiveness of the products must be used to hold the compounded products that are created.

5. Compounding of various substances, securing of all prescribed medications or devices, measuring dosage forms, collecting ingredients for sterile preparations, determining amounts of ingredients to be compounded, disposing of waste materials, packaging finished preparations, generating and affixing labels, storing all medications correctly.

Chapter 4

Fill in the Blank

1. brass
2. porcelain
3. liquids; semisoft
4. particle
5. 2.5
6. baths
7. Cylindrical; conical
8. straight; sloped
9. plastic; hard rubber
10. 5

Matching

1. F   2. D   3. C   4. E   5. B   6. A

Chapter 5

Multiple Choice

1. D   2. D   3. D   4. A   5. C
6. B   7. D   8. A   9. C   10. B

Fill in the Blank

1. base
2. single-phase
3. water
4. on top
5. cap; separated
6. 5; 000
7. pegboards; plates
8. trained

9. capsule
10. pipettes

Chapter 6

Multiple Choice

1. A   2. B   3. D   4. A
5. C   6. C   7. B   8. D
9. B   10. D

Fill in the Blank

1. computers
2. labeling
3. vaginal
4. 120
5. D
6. weight
7. unit
8. single dosage
9. spillage; evaporation
10. disposed

Chapter 7

Multiple Choice

1. D   2. B   3. C   4. D
5. A   6. C   7. D   8. B
9. C   10. A

Fill in the Blank

1. asepsis
2. hand washing
3. general cleaning; disinfecting
4. seconds
5. stainless steel
6. Grade A
7. chemotherapeutic
8. parenteral
9. year
10. 8 hours; dirty

Chapter 8

Multiple Choice

1. D   2. D   3. A   4. D   5. B

Matching

1. E   2. C   3. D   4. A   5. B

Fill in the Blank

1. ¼; 3
2. primary line
3. fluids; another
4. luer-lock
5. male
6. auxiliary
7. particles
8. wet; area
9. procedure
10. garments

Chapter 9

Multiple Choice

1. C	2. A	3. D	4. D	5. B
6. B	7. C	8. C	9. D	10. B

Fill in the Blank

1. multiple-dose
2. laminar-airflow hoods
3. 2003
4. three
5. syringe
6. container
7. 1 to 2
8. second
9. precipitation
10. 40

Chapter 10

Multiple Choice

1. A	2. D	3. D	4. D	5. C
6. B	7. D	8. A	9. D	10. D

Fill in the Blank

1. unit-dose
2. separately
3. access
4. cassette
5. laminar-airflow hoods
6. toxicity
7. "eyeball inventory"
8. inventory
9. price
10. shelf life

Chapter 11

Multiple Choice

1. A	2. B	3. D	4. C
5. D	6. A	7. C	8. D
9. B	10. D		

Fill in the Blank

1. ASHP
2. quality control
3. pharmacy; sterile
4. laminar-airflow
5. sterile
6. refrigerator
7. labeled
8. three
9. alcohol
10. Sterile products

Section I

Multiple Choice

1. D	2. B	3. B	4. C	5. C
6. B	7. D	8. B	9. A	10. A
11. C	12. D	13. D	14. B	15. C
16. B	17. D	18. B	19. D	20. D
21. A	22. B	23. D	24. A	25. D
26. A	27. D	28. C	29. C	30. C
31. B	32. C	33. D	34. A	35. A
36. C	37. D	38. A	39. B	40. D

Fill in the Blank

1. manufacturer's
2. hospital stay
3. formulation
4. osmosis
5. regulated; agencies
6. diagnosis; therapy
7. physical
8. emergency
9. contaminants
10. administering
11. avoid any errors
12. waste containers
13. unit-dose
14. mixing; assembling; packaging; labeling
15. virulence

Matching

    1. E   2. C   3. B   4. D   5. A

Section II

Multiple Choice

    1. A   2. C   3. D   4. C   5. C   6. A
    7. C   8. D   9. D   10. A   11. B   12. D
    13. A   14. B   15. C   16. D   17. A   18. A
    19. C   20. A   21. C   22. D   23. C   24. A
    25. C   26. B   27. D   28. C   29. D   30. A
    31. B   32. C   33. D   34. A   35. B   36. D
    37. C   38. B   39. C   40. B   41. D   42. A
    43. B   44. C   45. A   46. C   47. A   48. C
    49. D   50. A

Fill in the Blank

1. extemporaneous
2. state boards
3. 1 mg; 300 g
4. Isopropyl alcohol
5. magmas
6. gelatin
7. mortar; pestle
8. Wedgwood
9. pestle
10. dry
11. suspension
12. plastic; hard rubber
13. square
14. bristle
15. Tongs
16. glassine paper
17. Homogenizers
18. 6 months
19. pouch
20. 300

Matching

    1. H   2. E   3. C   4. G   5. D   6. F
    7. A   8. B

Section III

Multiple Choice

    1. B   2. D   3. C   4. B   5. D   6. B
    7. D   8. C   9. A   10. D   11. B   12. D
    13. C   14. B   15. C   16. B   17. D   18. A
    19. C   20. B   21. C   22. A   23. A   24. C
    25. A   26. B   27. D   28. C   29. D   30. C
    31. B   32. D   33. C   34. C   35. B   36. A
    37. C   38. A   39. D   40. C   41. B   42. B
    43. C   44. D   45. A   46. C   47. D   48. B
    49. A   50. D   51. D   52. C   53. D   54. B
    55. A   56. C   57. D   58. C   59. D   60. D

Matching

    1. K   2. E   3. L   4. D   5. H
    6. B   7. C   8. G   9. F   10. A

Fill in the Blank

1. manufacturer
2. abuse potential
3. toxicity
4. contamination
5. return forms
6. chemotherapeutic
7. time
8. laminar-airflow hoods
9. pairs
10. licensed
11. sterile compounding
12. laminar
13. shelf
14. sterile
15. 28 hours
16. infusion
17. unit
18. quality control
19. household bleach
20. colored band
21. hand washing
22. clean rooms
23. 250
24. *Journal*
25. vial
26. pumps; infusions
27. macronutrients
28. garb
29. infusion
30. additive

True or False

    1. T   2. F   3. T   4. F   5. F
    6. T   7. T   8. T   9. T   10. F
    11. T   12. F   13. T   14. F   15. T
    16. F   17. F   18. T   19. T   20. F

Glossary

A

Admix – Mix or blend.

Alum – Aluminum sulfate; used to help boost immune response, as an emetic, or as an astringent or styptic (both of which cause contraction).

Ambulatory care compounding – This type of compounding is designed for non-institutionalized patients; they may be outpatients or home-care patients.

Ampoule – A small glass container commonly used to hold hypodermic injection solutions or powders for reconstitution into these solutions; they often have tops that are designed to easily break off prior to use.

Anaphylaxis – An acute, severe, systemic hypersensitivity allergic reaction.

Asepsis – The process of inhibiting growth and multiplication of microorganisms.

Aseptic technique – Preparing and handling sterile products in a manner that prevents microbial contamination.

Audit – Examination or verification conducted to assure effectiveness and correctness.

Autoclave – High-heat, high-pressure device used to sterilize equipment.

B

Back-ordered – Temporarily unavailable from the supplier; also known as short.

Bacteria – Simple one-celled microbes that are named according to their shapes and arrangement; they cause infections throughout the body.

Barrier precautions – Precautions used to minimize the risk of exposure to blood and body fluids; this includes personal protective equipment.

Batch – A group of similarly prepared substances.

Batch-prepared prescriptions – Those in which multiple identical units are prepared in a single operation, in anticipation of the receipt of prescriptions.

Beyond-use date – A date for a sterile drug product calculated from the time it is compounded until it is administered to a patient.

Biohazard symbol – Symbols used to designate biologic materials that may be infective, and can possibly threaten humans or the environment.

Blister package – A type of medication packaging that features a hollow plastic/PVC portion containing the medication, which is backed by a paper or foil backing that peels off from the "blister" portion.

Bulk compounding formula record – Listing of ingredients and recipe for a specific medication formulation; also known as a master formula sheet.

C

Capsule – A solid dosage form featuring a drug contained inside an external shell.

Carts – Vehicles commonly used to move supplies and equipment in medical workplaces.

Cavitation – The rapid swelling and collapsing of microscopic bubbles.

Chart orders – A prescriber's instructions for diet, nursing care, laboratory tests, medications, and treatments for an inpatient.

Class A prescription balance – The most commonly used balance by pharmacists; it is a one- or two-pan torsion balance that may be digital (electronic weight sensing) or spring-based in design; the two-pan type requires the use of external weights for measurements exceeding 1 g.

Clean technique – Use of practices such as hand washing, general cleaning, and disinfection to reduce the presence of pathogenic microorganisms; also known as medical asepsis.

Cleaning – Physical removal of soil, blood, and debris from instruments and other items.

Compounding – The preparation, mixing, assembling, packaging, or labeling of a drug or device as the result of a practitioner's prescription drug order.

Compounding slab – A hard, non-absorbable flat surface used for the compounding of different medications or substances; usually made of ground glass.

Conical graduate – A container that resembles a cone—hence the name—with a wider top that tapers down to a thinner base; it has graduated markings for measuring liquids.

Conjunctiva – A thin, clear, moist membrane that coats the inner surfaces of the eyelids and the outer surface of the eyes.

Contamination – Containing unwanted substances or organisms.

Counter balance – A double-pan balance designed to weigh large quantities of bulk products.

Creams – Pharmaceutical preparations that combine oil with water, and are usually used topically.

Cylindrical graduate – A container that is cylindrical in shape, with the top being of the same circumference as the base; it also has graduated markings for measuring liquids.

D

Disinfection – Destruction of pathogenic microorganisms by exposure to chemicals or physical agents.

Disposable product – Intended to be used once for a specific patient, and then discarded.

Durable medical good – Intended for long-term use, though they are to be cleaned between each use.

E

Electronic balance – A scale that uses electronic components and digital readouts to calibrate the weighing of different substances; electronic balances are most frequently used now.

Elixirs – Liquid dosage forms that are sweetened, and contain alcohol and water.

Emulsion – A type of suspension that consists of two different liquids and an emulsifying agent (an emulsifier) that holds them together.

Engineering controls – Devices that isolate or remove the bloodborne pathogen hazard from the workplace.

Environment – A compounding environment consists of a separate area that is clean, neat, well-lit, and quiet; aseptic conditions are usually required.

Equipment – Compounding equipment includes clean air environments, electronic balances, ointment slabs, spatulas, mortars, pestles, electronic or manual capsule-making devices, glassware, and sterilization devices.

Ergonomic – The applied science of equipment design, intended to maximize productivity by reducing operator fatigue and discomfort.

Expiration date – A date, assigned by a drug's manufacturer, after which its stability and potency can no longer be guaranteed; also known as its beyond-use date.

Expiration dates – Estimated dates at which drugs are no longer at their effective potential; they are based on proper storage in approved containers away from such factors as heat and humidity.

Exposure control plan – A set of written procedures for the treatment of persons exposed to biohazards or similar chemically harmful materials.

F

Filter – A device used to separate certain elements or particles from a solution.

Flora – Microbial organisms occurring naturally in the body.

Forceps – Used to pick up prescription weights and ensure that oil is not deposited on the weight.

Formulas – Standards for compounding that ensure batch-to-batch consistency, documentable procedures, and proper preparation methods and ingredients.

G

Gauge – The size of the needle.

Gel – A jellylike substance commonly used for topical application that consists of particles mixed into a liquid, usually with an absorption base.

Geometric dilution – The mixing of a medication with an equal weight of a diluent, then an equivalent amount of diluent, until all the diluent is mixed in.

Glassine paper – Used underneath substances to be weighed to keep them from soiling balance pans; today, weighing boats are preferred over glassine paper.

H

Hazard communication plan – The application of warning labels that signify different types of hazardous chemicals.

Hazardous waste – A substance that is potentially damaging to living organisms and the environment.

Hospital pharmacy compounding – Compounding of drug products within a pharmacy that is located inside a hospital; it can provide better care and cost savings both to the hospital and to patients.

I

Infection – The invasion of the body by pathogenic microorganisms and their multiplication, which can lead to tissue damage and disease.

Infusion – The controlled flow of an intravenous medication into a patient.

Insufflation – A powdered medication blown into a nasal passage or ear canal.

Intermittent infusions – Small-volume parenterals.

Intravenous – Injected into the veins.

Intravenous (IV) bags – Pre-filled, sterile plastic bags used to contain intravenous solutions prior to administration.

Intravenous (IV) tubing – Plastic tubing used to transfer intravenous fluids from IV bags or bottles, through needles, into the body.

Invoice – Bill for goods received.

L

Legend drug – Another name for a prescription drug.

Levigate – To grind a powder into a smooth surface using moisture.

Liquid drugs – The most common form of compounded medications.

M

Magmas – Gels that have large particle sizes in a two-phase system.

Master formula sheet – Listing of ingredients and recipe for a specific medication formulation; also known as a bulk compounding formula record.

Material Data Safety Sheet (MSDS) – Written or printed material concerning a hazardous chemical that includes information on the chemical's identity, as well as physical and chemical characteristics.

Medical asepsis – Use of practices such as hand washing, general cleaning, and disinfection to reduce the presence of pathogenic microorganisms; also known as clean technique.

Medication administration record (MAR) – Documentation of the drug ordered, when it was given, how it was administered, the dosage given, and who gave it; used within the hospital setting.

Meniscus – The bottom portion of the concave surface of a liquid that is used to measure the volume of the liquid in a container such as a graduate.

Microbes – Minute life forms; especially disease-causing bacteria.

Microbiology – The branch of biology that studies microorganisms and their effects on humans.

Microorganisms – Minute life forms that are invisible to the naked eye; they include both free-living and parasitic life forms.

Mortar – A vessel with a rounded interior in which drugs or other substances are crushed by means of a pestle.

N

NDC number – A unique number identifying a drug product; it indicates the manufacturer's name, drug strength, dosage form, and package size.

Needles – Hollow devices commonly used to inject medications into the body, or to withdraw fluids from the body.

Nosocomial infection – Infection acquired in a hospital or institutional environment.

Nuclear pharmacy compounding – This type of compounding focuses on radioactive drugs (radiopharmaceuticals) that are used for diagnosis and therapy.

O

Occupational Safety and Health Administration (OSHA) – A Department of Labor agency that is responsible for ensuring safety at work and a healthful work environment.

Ointment – A highly viscous or semisolid substance used on the skin that may be referred to as an emollient or a salve.

Over-the-counter (OTC) – Medications that are deemed safe for use without the oversight of a physician.

P

Parenteral – Administration route other than through the digestive tract; most commonly refers to drugs administered intravenously.

Parenteral – Bypassing the skin and gastrointestinal tract; injected.

Paste – A semisolid pharmaceutical preparation that is intended for external use.

Perpetual inventory – Ongoing system of tracking of drugs received by and sold in the pharmacy.

Personal protective equipment (PPE) – Specialized clothing or equipment worn to protect against health and safety standards.

Pestle – An instrument in the shape of a rod with one end that is rounded and weighted; used for crushing and mixing substances in a mortar.

Pharmacy patient profile – A confidential record that contains medical and billing information, along with a list of medications received by the patient.

Physician's Desk Reference (PDR) – The standard medication reference book found in most medical offices; it lists most available medications.

Physician's order form – Documentation used in the hospital setting to order medications for a patient.

Piggyback – A second intravenous solution, usually of smaller volume than a primary IV, which is administered using a Y-site (or different type) of connection on the primary IV tubing; also known as a rider, and is abbreviated as "IVPB" (meaning "intravenous piggyback").

Pipette – Also spelled "pipet," this is a graduated tube (marked in mL) used to transport a certain volume of a liquid or gas.

Potentiation – Undesirable or desirable increasing or diminishing of another drug's actions.

Pouch package – A type of medication packaging that consists of clear or light-resistant plastic/PVC bags which are sealed with an adhesive.

Powder – A dosage form that may be used when a drug's stability or solubility is a concern; they are often mixed into foods or liquids.

Prescription – A physician's order for the preparation and administration of a drug or device for a patient.

R

Repackaging – The breaking down of bulk medications into smaller packages for specific use, such as unit-dose packages.

Reusable product – Intended for limited use, with cleaning taking place between each use.

Routine prescriptions – Those that pharmacists may expect to receive in the future on a routine basis; also called "maintenance prescriptions."

S

Sanitization – Cleaning the environment to reduce the number of pathogenic microorganisms.

Sharps – Any sharp medical equipment, including needles, catheters, and other equipment that may potentially cause injury during handling.

Shelf life – The length of time a drug product can be kept in stock before its contents are altered by age.

Sodium hypochlorite – The least expensive and most readily available chemical for cleaning surfaces; it is also known as ordinary household bleach.

Solution – A liquid dosage form containing active ingredients that are dissolved in a liquid solvent.

Solvent – A liquid vehicle used to dissolve active ingredients in a solution.

Stability – Duration of chemical, physical, or microbiological properties of a substance that may be affected by temperature, light exposure, and specific container types.

Standard precautions – A set of guidelines for infection control.

Suppositories – Semisolid dosage forms that may be inserted into the rectum, vagina, or urethra for localized or system effects.

Suspension – A liquid dosage form that contains solid drug particles floating in a liquid medium which are easy to compound, but physically unstable; suspensions must be shaken well before being administered.

Syringes – The parts of hypodermic needle assemblies used to contain medications prior to injection through the actual needle into the body, or to contain fluids withdrawn from the body.

T

Tablet – A solid dosage form that is made by compressing the powdered form of a drug and bulk filling material under high pressure.

Total parenteral nutrition (TPN) – Nutrition system involving the intravenous infusion of lipids, proteins, electrolytes, sugars, salts, vitamins, and essential elements directly into a vein.

Transmission – A passage or transfer, as of a disease from one individual to another.

Triturate – Reducing particle size within a mortar and pestle.

Triturated – Reduced to a fine powder by grinding.

Turbidity – Muddiness created by stirring up sediment or having foreign particles suspended.

Tyvek® – A type of material used in certain medication packages; it consists of a very strong and impervious spun polythene material.

U

Unit-dose – Systems that contain medication in a single-unit package intended for single-dose administration to a patient.

United States Pharmacopoeia/National Formulary – A list of drugs for which standards have been established by the government; it is recognized as the official list of drug standards, as enforced by the FDA.

V

Vaginal syringes – Applicators used to instill vaginal creams and gels directly into the vagina; they consist of applicators with plungers intended for one-time use.

Vasoconstrictor – Any substance that causes narrowing of the blood vessels.

Vials – Small glass bottles that are commonly sealed with rubber or cork stoppers and used to store medications prior to use.

Virus – A microorganism smaller than a bacterium, which cannot grow or reproduce apart from a living cell.

W

Work practice controls – Precautionary measures that are taken to reduce possible exposure to bloodborne pathogens by altering the way a procedure is performed.

References

Reference List

Buchanan, E. C., & Schneider, P. J. (2004). *Compounding Sterile Preparations* (2nd ed.). Bethesda, MD: American Society of Health-System Pharmacists.

DeLaune, S. C., & Ladner, P. K. (2006). *Fundamentals of Nursing: Standards and Practice* (3rd ed.). Albany, NY: Thomson/Delmar Learning.

Hegner, B. (2003). *Nursing Assistant* (9th ed.). Albany, NY: Thomson/Delmar Learning.

J. J. Keller & Associates Inc. (1997). *NIOSH Pocket Guide To Chemical Hazards: June 1997*. Neenah, WI: Author.

Moini, J. (2006). *Pharmaceutical Calculations for Pharmacy Technicians: A Worktext*. Albany, NY: Delmar Cengage Learning.

Moini, J. (2004). *The Pharmacy Technician: A Comprehensive Approach*. Albany, NY: Delmar Cengage Learning.

Palko, T., & Palko, H. (1998). *Glencoe Medical Laboratory Procedures* (2nd ed.). Dubuque, IA: Career Education.

Thompson, J. E., & Davidow, L. (2003). *A Practical Guide to Contemporary Pharmacy Practice* (2nd ed.). Philadelphia, PA: Lippincott Williams & Wilkins.

Wedding, M. E., & Toenjes, S. A. (1998). *Medical Laboratory Procedures* (2nd ed.). Philadelphia, PA: F. A. Davis Company.

Index

Note: Page numbers followed by an *f* refer to figures. Page numbers followed by *t* refer to tables.